The Healing Within:

Chiropractic Exposed!!!!

Yaphet L. Hill, D.C.

ISBN-10: 1481229184
ISBN-13: 978-1481229180

DEDICATION

To my loving Mother to whom which I owe my deepest and most sincere gratitude for my introduction to one of the most fulfilling professions.

CONTENTS

ACKNOWLEDGMENTS

I wish to personally thank the following people for their contributions to my inspiration and knowledge ana other help in creating this book: Three oj my closest friends Kermit, Parthina, and Robert for their support professionally as well as socially. My family Carl, Emma, ana Kenyatta for moral support ana for being instrumental in my growth as a person.

INTRODUCTION

Chiropractic, it seems that just the name alone raises an array of different perceptions of whether Chiropractic is a legitimate form of healthcare. Many questions are asked regarding the origins of Chiropractic and what exactly a Chiropractor does. The purpose of this book is to expose the benefits and science of Chiropractic.

Learning how to live a life centered in wellness gave great purpose to my publication, which serves as guide to achieve this lifestyle. I wanted a sensible summary of various medical conditions and how certain lifestyle choices can assist in the management of these conditions. These lifestyle choices, because some are naturopathic in origin can help you better understand the chiropractic way of life.

The main reason for writing this book is to inform you, the patient, that healthcare should be more pro-active than reactive. Waiting for symptoms to arise before you seek medical attention can be a detriment. Symptoms are generally the last to show and the first to go, when dealing with a disease process.. Early detection and treatment of any condition can prevent the conditions from manifesting into more complex situation.

So what can you expect from this book? A better understanding of how better life choices can improve your overall health. We as a culture are so inundated with thinking that in order for something to be effective it has to be complicated. Nothing could be further from the truth. If it's complicated idea chances are it won't be used in this publication. It's that simple.

This book is going to talk about things that are simple to do that can make a huge difference in your overall health. When setting goals and accomplishments, they must be perceived as being obtainable or we aren't going to even attempt them. The processes discussed in this book will be full of easy, useable processes that can make a world of a difference in your life.

We unfortunately live in society of instant gratification and sometimes we want to change certain aspects of our lives overnight. The truth is that we can change our *mind* overnight, but changing our body that quickly is not likely. Although conditions and symptoms may appear out of the blue, it often times it takes a lifetime for them to fully manifest. So if you want to change your health for the better, you must look at the healing factor differently. Look at it as an ongoing process that you begin today.

In order to get anything from the book first begin by opening your mind. They say the mind is like a parachute, and it won't work if it's not opened. You must have an open mind to try out new ideas, especially those actions that may not be as widely accepted by the mainstream population.

We as a society fear change. Because of this we continue down the path of reactive healthcare that has us to the condition of health that we currently experience. Reactive healthcare has been the method by which we mostly abide by, with the expectation of being cured by that "magic pill." Curiosity might very well be the help you need to bridge the gap from where you are to where you can be. Be curious with trying new things. Be open to new possibilities. Be open to becoming more health conscience. Although it might not seem to be "working at first," understand it may take a little time for your body to adapt to the subtle changes you've made. True healthcare is a lifestyle change and not merely popping a new set of pills to feel better. Life is a process. It is an experience. We must go through life with the courage that we will sometimes fall or sometimes fail. But, so what! All we do is just get back up. That is the key to success. Get back up when you fall.

Open your heart and open your mind and begin to explore the possibilities of a new life. The life I am talking about is a life with more energy, more vitality, and most of all, a life full of HEALTH.

TECHNOLOGICAL ADVANCES IN HEALTHCARE

Sure technology has had a great impact on healthcare. We see the evolution of the MRI's, x-ray, and ultrasound that allows us see into the body what we could only approximate before. In this book, however, you will learn about a technology that is so simple to use that it will blow you away. You will see the simplicity of health. Anyone trying to complicate health is trying to get you to be dependent on them so you rely on them solely, and you forget your own judgment.

That has been the problem within the healthcare system for some time. We have abided by the opinions of our healthcare professionals and their latest technologies, but it has brought us no more health than we expected. In the USA we in spend more money in healthcare than any other country in the world, yet according to the World Health Organization (WHO). The WHO reports that the U.S. ranks 37th out of 200 countries in terms of quality of individual health and wellness. To put that into perspective, Costa Rica is ranked 36th. Mediocre results from a country that spends more dollars on health care than any other country in the world is unacceptable.

What we are doing is simply not working. Innovation is at the heart of this book. No more complex strategies; we are going to get to simple, bare bones concepts that you can immediately use in your everyday life and that can truly make a difference in your life.

Break away from the old mindset and decide today for yourself that you are going to use a technology that will truly make a difference in your life. You deserve it, and those around you deserve someone who comes to the table alive, refreshed, energetic, and not just a partial representation of themselves. You deserve to reach the full you at your greatest potential! It should not be an option; this is your birthright.

Why do we need to think outside the box? This expression has been used for many years now and although it sounds cliché, it holds true more today than ever. We must change our paradigm from disease care, which we are clearly in, to a more preventative way of looking at health. It's the most cost effective way of taking care of our bodies.

This is not a new concept in other areas, so why should it be so underutilized when it comes to health? The automotive companies have known about it since cars were invented. They are well aware that if you give your car preventative care such as periodic tune ups and oil changes they will last longer. It's that simple.

So the key is to trim the fat from our healthcare. I believe the best way to do that is not to rely on symptoms. If you wait until there are symptoms, most often you are too late. You will learn more about this later in the book, but please keep that concept in mind.

The tests and processes we are using to determine health are not showing the consequences of our diets of ten years ago. It doesn't show what is going on with our arteries from the stand point of what the food we consume today is going to do to our arteries 5 or 10 years from now. Insanity has crippled this health care system, and we must do something about this now, before it's too late. If we continue at this rate in 50 years we have the unfortunate opportunity of bankrupting this country due to health care costs. HMO's and other insurance plans cost are increasing gradually, and it is predicted that within 5 – 10 years health care deductibles will reach an annual level of more than $5,000 per person. That is outrageous. We all can change this by approaching our own health in a preventative, proactive manner.

"THE GREATEST WEALTH IS HEALTH"

~VIRGIL

WHAT IS "HEALTH?"

~1~

If I were to ask you to define the term "health" What would be your answer? There is a general opinion and consensus that good health is: (1) feeling "fine," (2) when everything is working well, or (3) when there is an absence of pain.

All of these definitions are partially correct but are integral in the. Taber's medical dictionary defines health as, "A condition in which all functions of the body and mind are normally active." The World Health Organization defines health as a state of complete physical, mental, or social well-being and not merely the absence of disease or infirmity. So the next question to ask is how does one quantify health? In a sense then, health is equal to balance. How do you determine balance? What are the determining factors in the balancing equation? To answer this we must first ask, what comprises the overall scheme of health? Also, what kind of an overall gauge can be used to reflect back on the quality of health we experience or lack thereof?

In order to get to the fundamentals of good health you need to start at the cellular level. The balancing act begins there. You see the quality of your life is based on the quality of the life of your cells. Considering the fact that you are comprised of over 70 trillion cells, you can assume that when those cells are working optimally in perfect harmony with each other, you will have health. But again how does one quantify this?

Now if health equals balance, then we can state that the opposite of health, which is not disease, but rather "dis-ease" meaning a lack of balance or ease. It can also be said that the cells are not functioning correctly.

Raymond Francis, a chemist and graduate of MIT, believes through his research that there is only one reason in which disease is created. That reason is simply due to cells not functioning properly. When you think about that statement, it makes sense. Now there are only two reasons why cells do not function appropriately. They are:

1. Cells are not receiving proper nutrition and/or
2. Cells are not eliminating their toxicity produced by the normal functioning of the cell.

Now there are at the root many reasons why these cells can become dysfunctional. Those reasons are:

- Lack of appropriate levels of oxygen
- Lack of nutrients
- The inability to eliminate waste
- Improper nerve impulse to the cell

To begin to understand this process let us quickly visit the stages of health. When one is conceived, we are given as a birthright the ability to express health effortlessly. However if there is a disturbance in the intimate relationship between the nervous system and the rest of the body, you will lose your efficient ability to express health.

As we age, we experience the effects of the years initially only through a microscopic inspection. Long before we feel the effects of age, our cells are beginning to experience changes. Cells are beginning to replicate less efficiently, and then one day we transition from the anabolic phase of life, which means that sufficient cells are replacing those that have just died, to a phase of catabolic metabolism, in which we have more cells that are dying than are being replaced. When we enter the catabolic stage, we must do everything within our power to slow it down.

To better understand the process of health, it helps to understand the phases of health. The first phase is one of perfect balance or homeostasis. This is optimal health where everything is working the way it was designed to work. However, as we age, we begin to encounter emotional, physical, and chemical stresses in our lives to the point where we will enter into a phase of imbalance, lack of ease, or dis-ease. Health can easily be regained in this phase as long as we refocus our efforts on finding the cause of what brought us initially on that path of imbalance. If that is achieved, then we can regain a state of balance.

However, if this phase is not dealt with appropriately, then we enter into a phase of discomfort, and dis-ease. This phase can have with it associated levels of pain, but not in all cases. Sometime there are no visible or tangible symptoms. If we stay in this phase for any real amount of time, we begin to have dis-ease of more than one cell. It begins to affect thousands and thousands of cells, to the point of reaching into the body's tissues. Left further without a reversal of the dis-ease, then it enters into a larger group of tissues which would then be affecting organs. It then moves onto systems, and then ultimately it affects the entire being, and we then die.

[9]

I'm not proposing that we can live forever. I am however saying that 90% of our medical expense is spent during the last 10% of our lives. People are no longer dying of natural causes. The majority of deaths in this country are related to degenerative processes. When one can minimize that process one can live a longer, higher quality of life.

Therefore, the key to overall health is to correctly determine the appropriate factors involved in health. This means managing health at the cellular level. Health is a consequence of choices one has made or not made.

A DOCTOR'S APPROACH TO HEALTH

Here's a hypothetical situation, imagine going to a doctor when you had nothing wrong with you. Your blood pressure, your cholesterol, and your weight were appropriate for your age and height. During this visit you told the doctor that all you wanted to do was maintain this? Hopefully he or she would say, "great," but they may not be able to offer you much more in the way of maintenance than to say, "keep on doing whatever you are doing." The point here is that that kind of advice would only work for so long. That is because western medicine is at best designed for the early detection of disease, but not for the prevention.

How would you react if your mechanic that told you that all you need to do for your car is bring it in and have the oil changed when the car starts to give you problems? We all know what that would do, don't we? We know what the consequences of not getting an oil change on time does to our car, which incidentally we will only have for 10 years at best, and yet we don't always give our

[10]

bodies that we will hopefully have for many decades, the same kind of preventative care.

ANTIBIOTICS & DIS-EASE

Why do we put so little effort into maintaining our bodies? Probably because we are conditioned to believe that there is a magic pill that can solve all of our problems. Again no medicine has ever cured anyone. The body does the healing; it happens no other way.

The birth of medicine could be attributed to the time when Robert Koch postulated the germ theory in 1860. Once this discovery took place, it was therefore emphasized and widely believed that microbes were the cause of disease. It was also widely accepted that the key to health was to destroy those foreign enemies.

This theory has resulted in the overuse of antibiotics to the point that we are now dealing with super-strains of bacteria and viruses. These microbes are becoming more and more resistant to all of the antibiotics originally created to fight them off.

ALTERNATIVE HEALTH OPTIONS

Today people are becoming more and more aware of alternatives. They are sick and tired of being sick and tired and they want options. They want to know why they are sick or why they are feeling a certain way. They are sick and tired of hearing obscure explanations on what they have and why taking a "magic pill" will solve all their problems.

We are becoming more aware. In the United States in the year 2001 there were more visits to Alternative Health Care practitioners than traditional allopathic medical doctors. It may have started with the baby boomers who wanted to create and maintain health, not just mask their problems with drugs and surgery. We are not being attacked by the flu. We are not innocent victims being chosen by microbes. We are in fact creating the very environment for these bacteria and viruses to feast upon a body that is full of toxicity -- the perfect environment in which bacteria and viruses thrive.

Anyone can change their attitude and approach to health. If you continue to look at your body the same way you have in the past, you will continue to get what you have gotten in the past. However, if you want to change things, start with your mindset. You must prioritize your health as something that must be maintained and even improved, instead of something that is merely tolerated. In life, we consistently make time for things that we make a priority. It is important, therefore, to look at your health as top priority.

To make your health a priority you must realize that there are a variety of different choices we make daily that can be categorized into two broad areas: Doing things that are important and urgent; and doing things that are important and not urgent.

Everything in your life that adds meaning to your life and fulfillment to it, such as spending time with your family, spending time giving thanks to your creator, working out, eating the right foods, spending quality time with your significant other, are all under the category of things that are important but not urgent. In order for you to create the highest level of health possible, you must consistently focus on doing things in the area of health that are important for you.

The question to ask your self is, "What can I do today to start on a path of wellness?" I recommend that my patients make the changes that are very easy to do. For example, I had a patient who had not exercised in years. To get her back on track, I suggested that she try walking about 15 minutes a day 3 times a week. Of course that sounded very easy to do. Gradually that 15 minute walk turned into 20 minutes then 25 minutes. Next, she realized that the walking gave her more energy throughout the day and she began to sleep better. By the end of a month, she was up to a half hour of walking and began to inquire about adding light exercises to her regimen. She began to feel so good that the habit she has resurrected was one she intended on maintaining.

Once you create a habit, you can expand upon it, but you will set yourself up for failure if you start too big. The most important thing that I want you to get out of this chapter is the subtle consequences our choices have on our health. There are small decisions we make daily that can make the difference between being completely well or not.

If you would like to test out this theory for yourself, I have an assignment for you. First, get yourself a health journal. It can be any small notebook that you can keep with you. Next, write down the following on the inside cover or first page of your journal:

"I hereby grant myself permission to bring my health to the highest level I was meant to experience, by nurturing myself, by taking care of myself, and by forgiving myself as I would a loved one. I declare today, a day that I will never forget, for it is the day that my life and health was changed forever."

Your health journal should begin with a list of goals. These can categorized as physical, mental, and spiritual. You may want to eat better, so be specific, and list the types of foods you will avoid to obtain better health. If you want to learn a new skill or improve a relationship, list specific actions you can take and over which you have complete control. The more specific you are the more successful you will be.

Each day, record in your journal or notebook the small steps you have taken. Record even your setbacks and shortcomings because those will help you see the progress you are making over time.

HOW CAN CHIROPRACTIC CARE EFFECT YOUR HEALTH?

The biggest way Chiropractic can help you is by allowing one not to focus on symptoms, but rather on the body's ability to regain health. If you always chase symptoms, you will never truly regain your body's health potential. You will always be days or months away from your next symptom, and you will be focused on relieving those symptoms as quickly as possible.

Being under chiropractic care allows you to change your perception of going to the doctor only when there is a problem to going to the chiropractor because you don't want to have any problems in the future.

Where would we be if we had a health care system in which the doctors were only paid based on how healthy their patients are? Sounds insane or very theoretical? That's exactly what is happening in Japan. Doctor's get paid based on how healthy their patients are. It does not impress me whatsoever, when a doctor says that it's a good thing that you came in because we just found some major problems in you, and we need to go in immediately for a surgery. Problems like that just don't appear out of nowhere. It takes years and years for conditions to develop and get to that point. Again we have technology within the medical community that emphasizes early detection at best and very little, if any, prevention.

You can't just blame the doctors here either. It is the responsibility of each individual to care for themselves and to take action to prevent disease. It is the responsibility of every parent to see that their children are on a path of good, lifelong health through preventative care.

HOW CAN CHIROPRACTIC BE A STRATEGY TO ATTAIN HEALTH?

The science of chiropractic is in and of itself a fundamental strategy for good health. When you are under chiropractic care, you work to reduce any stress or strain around the spine which in turn could affect the body's ability to adapt to all that is thrown its way.

If there is any kind of interference within or surrounding the nervous system it causes dis-ease or creates a situation where you are not completely well. Often that interference can't be felt. There may no pain or pressure at all to tell you something isn't right. Rather the only thing you experience from this is the effects of it. Sadly, it may take months or even years for the symptoms to manifest themselves.

This might be easier to understand if you use the example of breast cancer. Did you know that it takes years to create enough density within the breast tissue in order to see a tumor growth via X-ray? By that time it may be too late.

Chiropractic does not emphasize waiting for something to go wrong, and then coming in as the hero to only remove the symptom, doing very little about the actual cause of the problem. It focuses on maintaining your natural state of wellness at an optimal level of existence, so that you are at the highest level neurologically speaking.

Think about it this way: if you applied the same rationale to your life in every aspect, would it make your life better or richer, or would it make it worse? If you applied the preventative model to your finances, what would it do? If you applied it to your relationship with your spouse, what would that do? All the areas of your life would see a marked improvement. You would no longer be waiting for things to get to the point of being urgent. You would be more proactive instead of reactive. You are prioritizing your health as being important while not waiting for a crisis to make changes.

HOW CHIROPRACTIC CAN CHANGE YOUR LIFE?

The system I propose is based on a true mind body approach that I call the IE technology – or Information and Empowerment. You see with information and empowerment, you can truly make a difference in your life. Here is a summary of the key factors needed to sustain health. More details are provided in the chapters on nutrition and exercise.

[16]

The first aspect of the system involves beliefs. You must first create the mental construct that will allow you to filter a reality with which you want to be congruent. In other words, you must believe in things that you want to have happen.

Next, is to understand the importance of exercise. You must exercise. It is not an option, and you can't justify not exercising because you already work hard at work, you already chase the kids around the house, and you already work in the garden. All of these activities are a good start to movement, but do not constitute a real workout. You must have a cardiovascular workout for health – one that challenges and works your heart. Remember your heart is a muscle and it needs to pump a lot of blood through your entire body every day for a very long time. You must challenge it so it can be as strong as possible.

The third aspect of this equation is the importance of breathing correctly. You must provide oxygen to the tissues of the body. If you don't, you will have problems because they will suffocate. Oxygen supplies and nourishes not only the lungs, but every cell within the body. The lungs are just the clearinghouse.

The fourth important factor is drinking water. This is necessary in order to flush out toxins from the body. After all your body is 75% water; not 75% coffee, or tea, or soda. These drinks just give you an illusion of energy. There is no sustaining power behind any of them, even though the caffeine addict may object to this statement.

The next fundamental truth relates to greens. Most people do not understand the magnitude of the importance of greens. Eating enough green, leafy vegetables each week is one of the most powerful things you can do for yourself. Think about this, to understand why plants are so necessary to good health. When plants are outside, they convert light into energy, in the process known as photosynthesis. Through this amazing process, we are able to literally consume energy through the plants.

Most importantly, you must consume some raw vegetables, or you are totally defeating the purpose. Raw plants contain the necessary enzymes that are often destroyed by over cooking. Enzymes are vital to good health.

The next nutrient that you need to have is antioxidants. Antioxidants allow you to minimize the ravaging effects of free radicals that are within us and increase in number as we age. Free radicals are produced in times of stress, during injury, or during chemical processes that are taking place due to the consumption of processed foods. Free radicals left to roam can cause damage right at the cellular level. Damaged cells lead to a lowered immune system and increase the likelihood of infection and disease.

The next dietary items you need to have are fats and oils. Fats are needed to assure that your body has sufficient levels of oil to make the cell membrane of the cell. This outer layer of the cell is made of a double layer called a biphospholipid layer.

The problem with fats and oils in the diet is that many of us consume too much or the wrong type of fats. According to researchers, the average person is deficient in correct oil consumption by up to 90%! That is staggering considering the connection between low levels of essential oils in our diets and cardiovascular disease and the resulting list of degenerative disorders. So, believe it or not, oils are by far the best preventative measure that you can take.

The last pro-active step you that you need to take is to maintain a healthy nervous system. Think about this for a moment. If you were consuming everything that I recommended, and yet your nervous system was not functioning properly, how would the brain tell the cells what to do with the nutrients it just received? How would the brain contact the cell to let it know when to remove waste?

Consider this research from a professor by the name of Professor Tzu. He claims that pressure put on a nerve with the weight of only a dime can interfere with normal transmission of impulse by up to 60%! It is staggering how little pressure it takes to reduce your body's own ability to send corrective, healing messages by so much.

"HEALTH IS NOT VALUED UNTIL SICKNESS COMES"

~THOMAS FULLER

The History of Chiropractic

~2~

Chiropractic is not a new concept or idea. It is quite the contrary. In the study of anatomy and physiology, the earliest physicians recognized the major role the spine played in health. Modern chiropractic, as a means of helping the body to heal itself and maintain wellness as it is practiced today, claims its first major historical breakthrough in the late 19th century. It is amazing to think that was only a little over 100 years ago.

As with ancient Chinese herbal medicine, acupuncture, homeopathy, or other "alternative medicines," chiropractic has a place in healthcare for those who are looking toward finding the cause of their pains and illnesses and treating them at the source, instead of covering up symptoms with a medicinal bandage. As a result, the history of chiropractic is still in the making as modern technologies along with time proven procedures work hand in hand to promote wellness.

ANCIENT HISTORY

Chinese and Greek writings dating back as far as 2700 B.C. imply that these ancient civilizations recognized the role of the spine in health. It was the Greek physician Hypocrites himself who is quoted as saying, "Get knowledge of the spine, for this is the requisite for many diseases."

Hypocrites wrote extensively about the spine. His recommended treatment for curvature of the spine, for example, stated:

"But the physicians, or some person who is strong, and not uninstructed, should apply the palm of one hand to the hump, and then, having laid the other hand upon the former, he should make pressure, attending whether this force should be applied directly downward, or toward the head, or toward the hips. This method of applying force is particularly safe."

Hypocrites noted throughout his writings that the physician should be knowledgeable of the spine. He remarks on procedures that worked and mechanisms that did not work so well. This exploration of the body gave physicians and other types of non-traditional healers a foundation from which to build as they discovered how nerves, carefully protected by this bone structure known as the vertebrae or spinal column, could be a key factor in how the body took care of itself.

Chiropractic, once referred to as "bone setting" continued to be practiced throughout the centuries up until the fall of the Roman Empire. Much of the learning and medical practices were lost during this dark period in history. Fortunately, some of the techniques were not lost and were handed down from one generation to the next. Variations for "bone setting" were used in Europe and Asia throughout the time period between the 11th and 15th centuries. Back walking was the name given to the act of walking on someone's back in order to cure certain ailments.

By the 1800s, a period of "enlightenment" was occurring in Europe. New medical procedures were being tried with some success. This however made medical doctors shun bone setting as an old fashioned and ineffective method of treatment. There was one famous surgeon who held onto the merit of bone

[22]

setting. In 1867, Sir James Paget gave credibility to spinal manipulation as a viable treatment in his article in the <u>British Medical Journal</u> entitled, *Cases That Bone Setting Cures.*

WHAT DOES "CHIROPRACTIC" MEAN?

The American Heritage Dictionary defines chiropractic (chi·ro·prac·tic) (noun) as:

"A system of therapy in which disease is considered the result of abnormal function of the nervous system. The method of treatment usually involves manipulation of the spinal column and other body structures."

Its word root is Greek from the words "chiro" meaning hand and "pracktikos" which means "practice." In short, it is the practice of using the hands.

This definition has been greatly expanded by the professional organizations and groups governing the practice of chiropractic. Chiropractic is often described with a few variations of the following:

"The science of locating and removing interference with the transmission or the expression of nerve force in the human body, by the correction of misalignments or subluxations of the bony articulations and adjacent structures, more especially those of the vertebra column and pelvis, for the purpose of restoring and maintaining health. X-ray and analytical instruments may be used for the purposes of chiropractic examinations."

It is this focus on the removal of interference with the nerves' abilities to complete the transmission that is the primary function of chiropractic today. It does not matter whether the misalignment is due to injury or just natural changes that happen to the spinal column through every day living. By removing the interference, optimum health is maintained.

As you will discover, however, throughout the profession of chiropractic., there are many different philosophies and practices that have been put into place by individual chiropractors that include much more than the adjustment of the spine. Since chiropractic can also be categorized as a lifestyle, there are many other practices that go along with spinal manipulations. Together, these take into account all aspects of wellness.

My personal chiropractic philosophy includes not only the adjustment of the spine but address muscular imbalances as well as nutritional deficits. This is because I see chiropractic as a profession of wholeness and in order to be effective the patient has to be treated as a "whole person."

CHIROPRACTIC CREDENTIALS – ARE CHIROPRACTORS DOCTORS?

If you have ever had any doubts about whether or not chiropractors are qualified to provide the important type of healthcare services rendered by the profession, this chapter should set your mind at ease. Doctors of Chiropractic (that is the official title once education and clinical training is completed), receive just about as much classroom education in anatomy and physiology and in biology and other sciences as medical doctors.

[24]

A student attending an accredited chiropractic college starts out with an average of four years of college level course work in a pre-medical, scientific field. Upon entering the college curriculum, the student begins the journey of another minimum 4,200 hours of classroom, laboratory, and clinical training. The majority of this time is spent in a clinical setting. It is very difficult to learn to adjust the spine and master the necessary amount of pressure and delicate balance of touch without hands-on experience. Once the classroom training has allowed the student to become knowledgeable on the functions and form of the body, the clinical experience prepares them to make accurate and precise adjustments. This kind of training also ranks Doctors of Chiropractic among the highest trained health care professionals. Here is a good comparison of the hours spent in training by a chiropractor and a medical student. There are many different numbers out there that vary from one medical school or chiropractic college to the next, so this chart summarizes the averages of several sources.

Subjects	Class Hours Chiropractic Students	Class Hours Medical Students
Anatomy	540	510
Chemistry	165	325
Diagnosis	630	325
Microbiology	120	115

Neurology	320	110
Obstetrics	60	150
Orthopedics	210	155
Pathology	360	400
Physiology	240	325
Psychiatry	60	145
Radiology	360	150
HOURS	3,065	2,710

ADDITIONALLY REQUIRED STUDIES

Chiropractic School	**Medical School**
Spinal Manipulation Nutrition Physiotherapy Advanced Radiology	Pharmacology Immunology General Surgery

Colleges of chiropractic that are accredited have obtained the approval of the Council on Chiropractic Education. This governing board is also recognized by the Secretary of the United States Department of Education. There are currently 22 accredited colleges of chiropractic and/or programs within the institutions around the world today. Those outside of the United States are also accredited by the local governing boards of the educational accreditation organizations for those countries.

BOARDS AND AGENCIES GOVERNING CHIROPRACTIC CARE

One of the most effective ways for any group of people to be monitored and to be held to a high standard while having a sense of accountability is to have them to be observed by their peers. Chiropractic has had a hard enough time gaining acceptance among some mainstream healthcare professionals, so it would be even more difficult if it were not for its strict requirements on licensing imposed by other chiropractors and the government.

The process of watching over the chiropractic profession begins with the education and training. Schools of Chiropractic can become accredited by an agency fully accepted and recognized by the U.S. Department of Education. Students graduate well-trained and prepared to practice chiropractic, but it doesn't stop there. Licensing in all 50 states in the United States, and by agencies around the world occurs to make sure Doctors of Chiropractic are trained to do what they say they can. Any type of field where a person's health and well-being can be impacted should be licensed and certified. Chiropractic is no exception.

National and state examinations must be taken to determine if a chiropractor is qualified to treat patients. There is a four-part test, and most states require passing scores on all sections. In addition, Doctors of Chiropractic in most states are required to participate in a certain number of continuing education hours each year in order to keep their current license.

[27]

State licensing agencies can be found at state divisions of occupational licensing and at boards of chiropractic examiners located regionally around the country. They are the watchdogs for the field so that only the top, most qualified chiropractors are able to work with patients.

Chiropractors are also part of a community of other chiropractors and can learn and further develop their skills through professional trade associations specific to chiropractic. Some of these organizations have programs recognized by the Council on Chiropractic Education that provide specific, specialized training in certain subcategories of chiropractic. Doctors of Chiropractic can become certified as specialists in orthopedics, neurology, occupational and industrial health, diagnostic testing, internal disorders, imaging, thermography, and sports injury. These specialties may help a patient decided on a potential chiropractor.

"THE DOCTOR OF THE FUTURE WILL GIVE NO MEDICINE BUT WILL INTEREST THEIR PATIENTS IN THE CARE OF THE HUMAN FRAME, IN DIET AND IN THE CAUSE AND PREVENTION OF DISEASE."

~THOMAS EDISON

CHOOSING THE RIGHT CHIROPRACTOR?

~3~

There is no question that who you choose as a chiropractor is just as personal as selecting a medical doctor. It is the same type of scrutiny you would give a new dentist or obstetrician when you look for someone to be an integral part of your overall wellness plan.

Since Doctors of Chiropractic are required to complete more than 4,200 hours of classroom, laboratory and clinical training, most come away from that training well prepared and qualified to care for you and your family. So the deciding factor for you may be more based on such subjective criteria as location, personality traits, gender, and practice policies. Most insurance companies today are recognizing the importance of preventative healthcare as well as the role of chiropractic. Most U.S. workers with heath insurance are covered to some degree for chiropractic visits. They pay their co-pays and visit the chiropractor as they would with any visit to a medical doctor. So cost is not usually a deciding factor in which chiropractor is right for you.

There are now more than 69,000 Doctors of Chiropractic world-wide and the numbers are quickly growing. Finding one close to home is also not a problem in most locales. The problem then becomes, deciding which of your neighborhood chiropractic offices meets your needs.

TYPES OF CHIROPRACTORS

Not all chiropractors are the same. There are in fact two general types of chiropractors with slightly differing views on how chiropractic fits into a plan for health and wellness.

[30]

There are some who view chiropractic as the only form of healthcare necessary for good health and in the treatment of all ailments. This group performs procedures to remove subluxations of the nerves in an effort to free the nerve signal to allow the body to heal itself by sending the proper information to the corresponding parts of the body. This type of chiropractor is referred to as a "straight chiropractor."

The second type of chiropractor is called a "mixer." In their practices they combine traditional straight chiropractic with other forms of natural healthcare. For example, mixers may employ practices such as electrical stimulations, massage, or hot-and-cold therapies to relieve pain and stimulate the body to heal and recuperate. A big part of a mixer's view on health is nutrition and exercise and their roles in maintaining a healthy spine and nervous system.

OTHER CHARACTERISTICS IN A CHIROPRACTOR

You may be looking for a woman Doctor of Chiropractic instead of a man. You may want someone who is especially good with children, if you plan to start your child's healthcare regimen off right with regular chiropractic care. There are other personality traits to consider since some people just get along with and feel more comfortable with certain types of people.

One trait you will very often find in a chiropractor is their focus on family. Many chiropractors are second or third generation Doctors of Chiropractic. It could very well be that chiropractic is America's number one family business, so to speak. Most likely, children of chiropractors become Doctors of Chiropractic themselves because they have been taught and realize the importance of chiropractic to overall health and well being. A child of a chiropractor will often relate to new patients that their first adjustment was administered just moments after birth to correct misalignments that may have occurred during the birthing process. This gentle fingering of an infant's spine will ensure all systems are go for the new life ahead.

The choice of which chiropractor to visit is a personal one. It is one that can be freely made on emotion, knowing that the governing National Board of Chiropractic Examiners, the Federation of Chiropractic Licensing Boards, and the Council on Chiropractic Education are constantly doing their jobs to make sure your practitioner is fully licensed and qualified to provide chiropractic care.

There are different types of chiropractors just like there are different types of medical doctors. In the medical field there are doctors that specialize in pediatrics, neurology, or endocrinology. The same holds true for chiropractors, but with some subtle differences.

All chiropractors receive the same general chiropractic education and training for the specialty of chiropractic – no matter what other course of study they may have pursued prior to the specialized chiropractic college curriculum. It is similar to a general practitioner gaining an education in all systems of the body and needing to have a general knowledge of all the correct functions so that when something is wrong they know just which specialist gets their referral.

Throughout the history of the world there have been "alternative" methods of health care. Ancient Chinese medicine, though in ancient times considered the only medicine, is now one alternative even many of those who frequent medical doctors also turn to. For some practitioners of chiropractic, the chiropractic form of health care is used instead of any other type of intervention. It is considered complete on its own. This is probably the most extreme and certainly the philosophy of "straight" practitioners.

A 1998 study (reference is found at the end of the book) of how the average person utilized the availability of chiropractic care indicated that the reasons for going to a chiropractor and the diagnoses from the visit were varied. The study by Hurwitz looked at the records of 5,000 chiropractic offices and found more than 130 different diagnoses. Most (13.7%) still dealt with sprains and strains of the neck and then other musculoskeletal systems. A small percentage of enlightened patients recognized chiropractic can do so much more. A total of 3.6% went for reasons such as headache, migraines, asthma, and myalgia and myositis.

Then on the on the other end of the spectrum is the Chiropractor that deals strictly with neck and back pain and injuries. These may be patients with chronic pain or those who have been in a car accident or people who one weekend just lifted a piece of furniture the wrong way. Their practice and procedures may be purely therapeutic and involve a finite number of treatments until the pain is better managed or eliminated.

Somewhere in the middle is where most chiropractors fit in today. These types of practices do deal with back pain and neck injuries, but also recognize that there are other illnesses, diseases, and every day aliments that can be treated and even prevented through regular manipulation and adjustment of the spine. To better understand how this type of chiropractor fits into a complete wellness program and integrates with the medical profession, first you need a better understanding of what is Chiropractic.

CHIROPRACTIC PRINCIPLES AND PHILOSOPHIES

What has really undermined the well being of our society has been an attitude of suppression versus stimulation. So, just what is this concept of suppression versus stimulation and what does it mean in terms of your own personal healthcare?

As a society we are focused on suppressing the symptom. We focus on getting rid of the cold by taking this or that to knock the cough, or get rid of the headache. We take an antibiotic to get rid of the bacteria that we have in us creating our ailments. The sad truth is that the more we use the medicine, the more dependent we will become on those medicines to create a normal life.

Suppression alone is not the answer. We must learn how to re-awaken the power of the healing capacity that we have deep within us all. By focusing on what you want, it is easier to get a much clearer understanding that you are creating something that you want. You don't want to just get rid of this pain; the real goal it to be healthy. Those two concepts are radically different, yet people overlook this difference all the time. Ignorance regarding this matter is going to destroy your health.

If you think that things are just going to get better on their own, without being proactive, you'll figure out eventually that concept doesn't work either. The sad truth is that 37% of people who die of a heart attack die without a symptom, except death itself. These are people that just got a check up, felt fine, got a clean bill of health and then maybe they went for a run, and dropped dead. Something was evidently if not obviously wrong.

We know that in cancer treatment, if we just focus on the suppression of the cancer, without the stimulation of the body's defensive capacity, we are going to severely compromise the person's ability to recover from the treatments. Sometimes just the treatment of the disease is what causes the patient to die in the end.

I don't want you to think that I'm trying to put down the medical profession. I know they are doing the best they can to provide the best care possible. But the truth must be told. What we are doing in our health care system is not working. It is not the first and best choice in maintaining health or even treating disease. It's not even close.

There are many terms used in chiropractic that may not be familiar to the lay person; terms such as *subluxation* or *innate intelligence*. These specific principles are extremely important and foundations upon which many other theories and practices within chiropractic are built.

Here we can look at the meaning of some of the key ideas found within chiropractic philosophy. You will also see now they are implemented and applied today

Innate Intelligence

The chiropractic way of thinking takes into account something that is called "innate intelligence." What this means in a nutshell is that the human body is completely self-sufficient in how it functions. The body automatically knows when to take a breath or increase the heart rate when more oxygen is needed. It

[35]

sends off a signal when it needs food or water. The body responds to a viral or bacterial infection by heating up in the form of a fever to burn away the foreign invader. It does all of this because the brain can automatically send signals without some external intervention.

The brain and nervous system as a whole is able to function whether we are awake or asleep. It knows what it needs and what to do about that need all on its own. The miraculous part of it all is that we are born with this innate intelligence. However, even from the beginning, from the process of birth, interference can get in the way of the free flow of the intelligence data needed to make the body perform optimally.

What is a Subluxation?

Since every organ in the body relies upon innate intelligence to function, the blocking of the free flow causes problems. It can show up as aches and pains – more signals that something isn't quite right -- or it can appear over time as illness and disease. This blockage or interference has a name within the chiropractic community called "subluxation" or nerve interference. Subluxation is also starting to have some recognition as a valid cause of illness within the medical profession as a whole. For the chiropractor, the subluxation is synonymous with "dis-ease" meaning there is a state of un-ease or lack of complete and proper function due to the blocked messages sent through the nerves.

The spinal column is the primary shield the body has to protect the spinal cord and the nerves. If it is in perfect form and alignment, the messages go about the body unhindered. Rarely does the body stay in this perfect state. We "tweak" our backbone doing any number of everyday activities, even during sleep. It could take months or years before any noticeable dis-ease occurs unless there is some major trauma to the spine. Even these seemingly minor misalignments can distort a perfectly clear message from transmitting to the organs it needs to visit. This is subluxation. The cure or solution is to open up that channel once again and let the signals flow freely. This is what chiropractic is all about.

Subluxation in a broader sense can refer not just to nerve signals and messages but any disruption of any spinal joint's function. This can be neurological or chemical. A subluxation can refer to interference with hormones or the mechanical or structural make up of the spine's function. Depending on the chiropractor that you work with, there can be slightly different interpretations of what a subluxation really is. Most chiropractors however will agree that it is a tangible inference in complete wellness.

To correct a subluxation the only known effect way is to get a chiropractic adjustment. Chiropractors are trained in removing the nerve interference through the gentle application of force to specific areas of the spine.

CHIROPRACTIC CARE FOR SUBLUXATIONS

The role of chiropractic is to find and correct subluxations. There are a few different ways that chiropractors go about doing this. The "old fashioned" way is still one of the best methods for detecting a misalignment of the spine. This is done through hands-on touch of the spine to feel for misaligned vertebrae that may be blocking signals. This sense of touch is highly developed in the chiropractor. Years of hand-on clinical training enable him or her to literally feel for mis-alignments that could be blocking the free flow of nerve signals. However, even as well developed as this special sense of touch is chiropractors today also rely on many other medical devices and advances in medical technology to help create an even more complete picture of what is happening within the body.

Another method of creating an image of the spine is through X-ray. All chiropractic colleges have extensive course work and practical experience in interpreting an X-ray for possible subluxation. The two methods used together, give the Doctor of Chiropractic a good overall picture of the spinal situation for the patient.

Some subluxations are easier to pinpoint than others. For example, if a patient comes to the office complaining of a pain shooting down their leg, it is fairly easy to locate the vertebra which is probably causing the "pinched" nerve. In reality, it may be that there are several vertebrae misaligned, and only the one responsible for protecting nerves to the legs is pressing on the actual nerve.

In other situations the subluxation may not be as obvious to the average person, but it is to the chiropractor. Each vertebra in the spinal column has a bundle of nerves that protrude. Each nerve, the wire if you will to send the messages, is appointed to a different organ or system in the body. So if a patient comes into the office complaining of chronic stomach aches, then it may be the nerves coming from the T6 (this is the 6th Thoracic vertebrae) in the mid-back are being blocked in some way by the vertebrae intended to protect them.

Dr. R.L. Hartman developed the spinal chart that shows the effects of specific vertebral subluxations on various systems and organs of the body. The table here summarizes and outlines so of the conditions or ailments that could be experienced from pinched nerves or areas of subluxation. It is not intended to be

[38]

a final diagnostic subluxation finder, but a good tool for examining which nerves may be affected by spinal changes. It helps the chiropractor know where to start after listening to the complete history given by the patient including any symptoms they are experiencing.

*CORRESPONDING VERTEBRAE & NERVES TO SYMPTOMS & CONDITIONS *

Cervical Spine	Parts of the Body Related to Corresponding Nerves	Symptoms or Conditions Possibly Resulting from Subluxation
C1	Head, Brain, Face, Pituitary gland, Inner and Middle ear, Blood flow to this region	Headaches, mental conditions, nervousness, dizziness, high blood pressure
C2	Eyes, Sinuses, Auditory and Optical nerves, Tongue, Forehead	Sinus and allergy problems, deafness, blindness
C3	Face bones, Teeth	Acne, eczema
C4	Nose, Mouth, mucous membranes	Hay fever, post nasal drip, infections in adenoids
C5	Neck glands and Vocal cords	Sore throats and laryngitis

[39]

C6	Muscles and glands in the neck, Tonsils	Tonsillitis, cough, croup, pain in neck and upper arm
C7	Thyroid gland, Elbows	Bursitis, tendonitis, over or under active thyroid

*CORRESPONDING VERTEBRAE & NERVES TO SYMPTOMS & CONDITIONS *

Thoracic Spine	Parts of the Body Related to Corresponding Nerves	Symptoms or Conditions Possibly Resulting from Subluxation
T1	Forearms, Wrists, Hands, Fingers	Pain in these regions and breathing problems, asthma
T2	Heart valves and Coronary arteries	Heart conditions and Chest pain
T3	Lungs, Chest, Breast	Bronchitis, pneumonia, congestion
T4	Gall bladder	All conditions of gall bladder including jaundice, shingles
T5	Liver, Blood	Liver conditions, low blood pressure, arthritis, anemia

T6	Stomach	Gastrointestinal problems, heart burn, indigestion
T7	Pancreas	Diabetes and hypoglycemia
T8	Spleen and Diaphragm	Serious infections and hic-ups
T9	Adrenal glands	Anemia, hair loss, obesity, allergies
T10	Kidneys	Fatigue, kidney malfunction
T11	Kidneys and Urethras	Skin conditions
T12	Lymph nodes, Fallopian tubes, Small intestines	Rheumatism, infertility, gas pains

*CORRESPONDING VERTEBRAE & NERVES TO SYMPTOMS & CONDITIONS *

Lumbar Spine	Parts of the Body Related to Corresponding Nerves	Symptoms or Conditions Possibly Resulting from Subluxation
L1	Large intestines, Colon	Diarrhea, constipation, hernias, colitis
L2	Appendix, Upper leg	Appendicitis, varicose

		veins
L3	Ovaries, Uterus, Testicles, Bladder, knee	Menstrual problems, impotence, bed wetting, knee pain
L4	Prostate, Lower back, Sciatic nerve	Painful or frequent urination, sciatica, backaches
L5	Lower legs, ankles, feet, toes	Poor circulation, leg Cramps, foot and ankle swelling and pain
Sacrum	Hips, buttocks	Spinal curvatures
Coccyx	Rectum, Anus	Hemorrhoids, pain while sitting

*(Table is a only partial listing and summarization of items contained on Dr. Hartman's Spinal Nerve Chart)

WHAT TO EXPECT DURING YOUR VISIT TO THE CHIROPRACTOR

If you are new to the wonder of chiropractic, you may be a little unsure about what to expect. Is there going to be some massage-like table slab where I lay down to have someone pound my back and crack my spine? Do I have to get undressed? Is there anyone else in the room with me during an examination or adjustment? These are all very good questions, that left unanswered could dissuade someone from visiting a chiropractor.

[42]

You may be surprised to know that a visit to the chiropractor is one of the most relaxing and comfortable type of health care visits – and I can almost guarantee it hurts less than going to the dentist: physically, emotionally and financially.

When you enter most chiropractor offices, you will be greeted by a warm receptionist (in some cases the doctor) ready to answer your questions and get some information from you. You will complete some paperwork on you health history and your insurance company so that they can be billed directly.

Rarely on your first visit, will you have any kind of adjustment or manipulation to your spinal column. This is a time for gathering information, including a comprehensive medical history, and for the chiropractor to really listen to what concerns you. It is a time to establish trust, make you comfortable, and discuss what possible therapy could benefit you.

Next, you may be asked to schedule a series of visits where X-rays, mobility tests, and other diagnostic testing can be completed. If there is acute pain, you may begin testing to expedite treatment in order to bring you more immediate relief.

"EVERY PATIENT CARRIES HERS OR HIS OWN DOCTOR INSIDE"

~ALBERT SCHWEITZE

Diagnostic Methods Used in Chiropractic

~4~

A typical patient evaluation and history taking is similar to that with traditional medicine. Chiropractors are trained to take histories and also to use diagnostic tools that will narrow down and differentiate between problems that can manifest similar symptoms.

Some of the standard tests used in chiropractic are orthopedic and neurological in nature. This means X-rays, ultrasound, and range of motion and mobility analysis.

There is also a hands-on analysis where a trained chiropractor is able to feel obvious misalignments in the spine. They are able to tell through touch when vertebrae have shifted to the point where there is interference with the neurological signals transmitted by the radiating nerves.

There are also some cutting edge technological advancements brought to light by the growing field of chiropractic. Working with the tried and true instrumentation and the newest technology allows chiropractors to get a more complete picture of the situation before recommending and beginning any kind of treatment.

Subluxation Stations

There is a kind of instrument used in chiropractic that can offer a complete look and analysis of where and what kind of subluxation is taking place in the patient. It uses a static surface electromyogram (sEMG) to measure

[45]

electrical activity and then create a color map of sorts of just where the nerve interference is taking place.

The colorful illustration is the result of what kind of electrical activity is taking place in the muscles around the spine. It measures paraspinal infrared temperature to automatically measure range of motion. Pain thresholds can also be measured along the spine with a subluxation station.

Thermal Imaging Instruments

Infrared imaging is used to view changes in temperature where soft-tissue injuries may have occurred. It also is able to measure increases in pain and then treat these areas with infrared light therapy which increases blood circulation to the area. It even has the ability to stimulate cellular and nerve function painlessly.

A process called Computerized Infrared Thermography (CIT) is also implemented through a handheld paraspinal scanner. One such instrument has been developed by Titronics Research and Development in Iowa, City, IA. The device scans and generates graphs that can be laid one over the other for analysis and comparison.

The Nervo-Scope

This instrument developed by the Virginia-based company, Electronic Development Labs, is used both before and after the chiropractor makes any adjustments to the patient's spine. Before the manipulation the scope makes an assessment of temperature readings taken along the spine. Following the adjustment, the readings are again recorded to measure the difference. This allows the chiropractor to see how much of a reduction in subluxation has occurred.

The Myogauge

This trademarked instrument created by the Myogauge Corp. in Deer Park, NY, primarily measures range of motion and isometric muscle strength for any part of the body. The systems are highly customized, so each practitioner can add the accessories that best serve their patients. The computerized system documents results from digitally measuring the amount of force created by the patient's movements.

Regional Spinal Testing

There are instruments used in chiropractic that focus on the various regions of the spinal column which measure and record such results as temperature and the waveform created by the spine. One such instrument is the Pro-Adjuster from Pro-Solutions of McMurray, PA. The Pro-Adjuster taps each segment of the spine to gather its objective data.

Other instruments used in spinal screening incorporate bilateral weight and postural evaluations. This is true of the Rapid Posture Imaging system (SAM) developed by the S.A.M. Company of Henderson, NV.

The reason for explaining the complex technology that is associated with chiropractic diagnosis is to illustrate for you the advances that have been made. A visit to the chiropractor is not a bone-cracking session based on hit or miss adjustments.

The spine is one of the most important, if not THE most important system in the body.   No legitimate, well-trained chiropractor is going to proceed with manipulations blindly.   There is constantly emerging and extremely sophisticated instrumentation and diagnostic tools available to make educated, pinpointed adjustments and then document the progress.

"NATURAL FORCES WITHIN US ARE THE TRUE

HEALERS OF DISEASE."

~HIPPOCRATES

SPINAL MANIPULATIONS AND ADJUSTMENTS

~5~

After the diagnostic stage of a visit to the chiropractor, there is the treatment phase of patient care. This is the hands-on physical part of the chiropractic visit. There is one final diagnostic stage that takes place before any actual spinal manipulation or adjustment and that is the spinal palpation. This is a hands-on test that uses touch to determine changes or irregularities in the tissue between the vertebrae and along the spine.

Spinal palpation can be either static or motion palpation. In static palpation the touch is done while the patient is still. Mostly this tests for sensitivity or pain and can detect swelling. It is a tactile diagnostic method used along with the visual images taken from X-rays and other imaging tests.

Motion palpation does just what the term implies – measures motion. There is a degree of motion that can occur in joints and along the spine, and then there is the end play. End play is the absolute end of the range of motion – that one bit more of flexibility after the natural stopping point in the range of motion. The degree of end play, with or without pain, is a useful diagnostic piece of data to have before any adjustments.

MANIPULATIONS TO REMOVE SUBLUXATION

Manipulating the spine through small and gentle movement of the vertebrae is the most effective way of elimination subluxation. Subluxation prevents the nerves from sending a clear, uninterrupted signal from the spinal column, which over time leads to illness and disease.

In chiropractic the term disease is actually broken down as dis-ease. This implies that there is a reduction in wellness, instead of the medical term which means more of a chronic or life-threatening illness. There is a fine distinction, but with chiropractic, the overall wellness and wholeness of the body are central to allowing the body to be the best it can naturally be. This state of being returned to a completely well and balanced state is known as "homeostasis."

THAT "POPPING" SOUND

Even though the bones are being gently adjusted and moved, there isn't any jerking or cracking, as some images of chiropractic may conjure up. The "popping" sound many people hear during an adjustment is called "cavitation." The sound is actually the release of nitrogen gases from the synovial fluid in the joint and is painless and harmless. It is a reaction that allows tissue to move freely and releases toxins from the body.

TYPES OF ADJUSTMENTS

Spinal adjustment in the early days of chiropractic involved almost all hands-on movement of the vertebrae to release the subluxation. The amount of pressure, angle of the movement and position of the hands were the primary methods for varying the affects of the adjustment.

Today during an adjustment, misalignments are corrected through both hands-on techniques and the use of instruments. Both techniques are effective in their main objective which is to return vertebrae to their proper positions and function. Most chiropractors today use many different techniques to realign the vertebrae. Some are done strictly by hand, while others employ such instruments as an activator which is a rubber tipped handheld instrument. The following lists some of the more common techniques. When performing these adjustments on children, either one hand or a couple of fingers would be used in place of the whole palm to adjust for their smaller size. Finger manipulations are done even on infants just a few minutes old.

Kinesiology

Kinesiology focuses on the muscles around the bones as well as the vertebrae themselves. Muscles related to the specific vertebrae are balanced through special procedures. This helps keep adjustments of the spine in place when the attached muscles are performing optimally.

Table Adjustments

This may be the most familiar of adjustment techniques, even to those who are new to chiropractic or who may have a preconceived idea about what a visit to the chiropractor may be like. During a table adjustment, the patient lies down on a special table. Quick thrusts are applied to a specific area of the spine. Simultaneous with the thrust, the table drops slightly. This is a gentler method than the straight manual adjustment. Less pressure is needed to get the spine to move.

Toggle Drop

A toggle drop also uses quick thrusts. The hands are crossed and applied to the problem point on the spine. It is a method that is extremely effective in improving the vertebral joints mobility.

Lumbar Roll

With the lumbar roll, a patient is placed on their side. This is effective in focusing in on one specific vertebra out of alignment. Again, quick thrusts are applied to the single vertebra.

Instrumental Adjustments

An instrument adjustment begins with the patient lying face down on the table. A spring-loaded instrument is activated to provide a very gentle movement of the vertebrae. This technique is gentle enough for children.

THE ROOT OF ALL HEALTH IS IN THE BRAIN. THE TRUNK OF IT IS IN EMOTION. THE BRANCHES AND LEAVES ARE THE BODY. THE FLOWER OF HEALTH, BLOOMS WHEN ALL PARTS WORK TOGETHER."

~KURDISH SAYIN

CENTRAL TO GOOD HEALTH: THE NERVOUS SYSTEM

~6~

When we were first conceived, the first thing created in all of us was the brain. Next, it was carefully encased in a bony hard substance called the cranium. Afterwards, the spinal cord, an extension of the brain was created, and that too was encased in a protective layer called the vertebrae or spinal column.

The next part to be developed in-utero was the spinal nerve roots, which are extensions of the spinal cord. Ultimately, those spinal nerve roots create spinal nerves which are surrounded by embryonic tissue. The brain is then stimulated by the embryonic tissue via the super highway called the nervous system. It was then and only then, that the other systems in the body developed.

You see the nervous system is what controls all the systems in the body. If you were to look up nervous system in the Webster's Dictionary, you would find it defined as the following: "The master control system of the body that controls all other systems of the body."

The nervous system consists of three different areas. The first is the brain. It is the originator of the messages that are needed to be distributed to all the cells, tissues, organs, and systems of the body.

The second part of the nervous system is the spinal cord. Think of it as the super highway of the nervous system. It is a complex system which has routes to every aspect of our body.

The third part of the nervous system is the spinal nerve. Think of this as an exit off the main highway. Without these exits, you can never really get to a specific destination.

The brain weighs only 3 pounds. It needs only the energy of a 10 watt bulb, yet the functions of the brain are truly staggering. The brain is so complete and complex in its function that you would need two buildings the size of the Empire State Building to house today's technology that would rival the power of the brain.

Let me explain further. The brain can perform billions of operations simultaneously. Billions! A computer can only perform one task at a time. A computer can perform the task at astounding speeds, but it can only perform one function at a time. Therefore, in order to have the computer be able to replicate the full capacity of the nervous system, you would need a massive system enabling the computer to perform complex tasks; billions of them at the same time. That is why the nervous system is called the master control system of the body. It controls all other systems. Without it, you could not survive.

Here is another way to emphasize the importance of the nervous system. If you cut the nerve to the lungs, how would the lung know what to do? Think of the lung as an appliance, and the spinal cord is the circuit. If the circuit breaker isn't allowing energy to flow into the outlet that supplies the appliance, the appliance is not going to work. It's the same with the cells, tissues, organs, and systems of the body.

THE WORKINGS OF THE NERVOUS SYSTEM

Intelligence flows through every cell in the body. This intelligence is referred to by chiropractors as Innate Intelligence. Without this intelligence, there would be no order and no divine collaboration within our body.

There is an internal divine guidance that guides all the functions of the body. It knows exactly what substance to produce at the exact time needed. The neuronal connections within our body are truly staggering. In the brain alone, there are more possible connections than there are possible combinations of phone lines within the Unites States. Just imagine that number!

So what prevents our body from doing its thing? What prevents this splendid orchestra from playing its tune called health?

Interference with the nervous system can have serious complications. Think about this for a moment. If I'm on a phone and I'm giving you very detailed instructions on how to get from point A to point B, and all of a sudden your phone begins to break up, will you be able to accurately get the directions you need to get to your destination? Now, this is not because you are incompetent. It is simply due to the fact that there was a break in your communication with me.

The key is to maintain 100 % communication within every aspect of the body. The researchers are just beginning to understand that there are mechanisms within our body that are trying to communicate something very important. One example is the fever. At first fever was regarded as something that needed to be stopped. We now know that it is designed to throw off the foreign invaders.

How did we react to fevers just 10 years ago? We pushed fever reducing substances down our children's throats, and we bought into it. There are so many examples of this type of message scrambling that we do to ourselves, be it emotionally, physically, nutritionally, etc. Misunderstandings take place all the time. That is why I'm writing this book -- to at least give you a basic understanding of your body and what you can do immediately to bring it the next level. You have a very sophisticated body which needs a sophisticated understanding on how to provide it with the essential care it needs.

If the entire nervous system is fully functioning and fully interactive, with all the cells, tissues, organs, and other systems in the body, then the body can effectively and efficiently respond appropriately to dangerous conditions in the body. However, if the nervous system is not functioning properly, then you will find that it will create an imbalance, or lack of ease also called dis-ease.

The mindset that we have in regards to our bodies must be changed. Do we just get by in a world that is cruel, or is life a miracle, and the body that I am in the temple of my soul? Do we have reverence for our bodies? Again this book is a wakeup call for you to realize that there is so much in all of us to stimulate health -- so much potential. Unfortunately, most of the time, through ignorance, the body is just wasted away.

In coming chapters you will realize that our bodies can be the most amazing source of super immuno-stimulation and yet it can also be the greatest source of disease creation. The great researcher Gary Null, has advocated that health can be broken down into 25% nutrition, 25% exercising, and a whopping 50% mental attitude. If we have certain expectations and we believe them with certainty, those expectations will manifest in the physical world. In other words, you truly become what you think about, good or bad. What we must remember is that the intelligence that created us at conception still flows through every cell in our body today, and we must honor that.

I tell my patients that the body is providing us with signals, and we cannot ignore those signals. Again, I will stress one thing; I or any other chiropractor, doctor or naturopath does not cure anything or anyone! The body does the curing. Think about it, you see all these doctors that boast about their achievements with patients, yet if they truly understood the innate intelligence that flows through us all, he or she would humbly become obedient to that intelligence and do everything they could to align themselves with the principles of health.

The body can either be used in its amazing splendor or it can be abused, and if it is abused, you will suffer with the consequences of natural law. So if we are to attain incredible levels of health, we must first start with an equivalent level of gratitude for our body and respect for it. When you realize that you have a choice, to make this life what you want of it, to carve out of life what you want, to create a magical life full of passion, vibrancy, and possibility, then you must be grateful for what you have. Think about it. There are so many things for which you can and should be grateful. The body that you are in right now is doing everything it can to support you at this very moment. It is there to serve you. So today I want you to decide that from now on, you will no longer look at your body as something that deserves a candy bar or a soda. Think of it as one of the finest, exotic cars in the world, one that deserves and should receive only the best fuel.

If you owned a $100,000 race horse, you would train it constantly. You would feed it the best food possible. Why? Because you paid all that money and you expect to get a return on your investment. Well what do you suppose you and your health are worth? How much would you be willing to pay for a liver transplant? How much for a kidney transplant? How much for a heart transplant? How much for your hearing? How much for your vision? Can you now see how valuable and priceless you really are?

Realize that you are a gift from your creator, and that you are here for a reason. That you are here not to be a wandering generality, but a meaningful specific, a person destined to achieve something worthwhile. You can't attain your heart's desires without the spark of energy derived from a true level of health and well being. Begin today with a new appreciation that your life demands true energy, not just bouts of it. It deserves a level of health that rivals the idea you once thought of as acceptable.

"THE PHYSICIAN WHO TEACHES PEOPLE TO SUSTAIN THEIR HEALTH IS THE SUPERIOR PHYSICIAN. THE PHYSICIAN WHO WANTS TO TREAT PEOPLE UNTIL AFTER HEALTH IS LOST IS CONSIDERED TO BE INFERIOR."

~AUTHOR UNKNOWN

THE SPINE

~7~

The primary component to chiropractic is, of course, the spine. It is the spine, which for the sake of our discussion is made up of the spinal cord and vertebrae that is central to the science of chiropractic.

By giving you a little anatomy lesson on the spine, it will help you understand how and why chiropractic makes so much sense to those of us who have adopted this practice as our lifelong vocation.

The spinal column is a row of bones that encircle the spinal cord. The spinal cord is the central component of the central nervous system which transmits signals throughout the body. Some people assume that the spinal cord and nerves only transmit signals about touch and pain.

It is believed that the nerves signal the brain when you touch something hot, pain then registers in the brain, and you quickly remove your hand from the iron. This much is true, but there is so much more information that the nervous system communicates to the brain and other organs in the body.

In chiropractic it is known that every area of the body is supplied with information that comes from the nerves. When there is no static, if you will, what chiropractors refer to as subluxation in the message transmitted, every organ can function at its fullest capacity. That is the number one purpose of chiropractic – to remove static from the message signals and open the channels for the body to mend and heal using its own innate intelligence.

REGIONS OF THE SPINE

The spine can be broken down into three key regions. There is the **cervical spine**, **thoracic spine**, and **lumbar spine**. There is also a fourth area referred to as the **sacral region**. The sacral region, however, only has two bones: the sacrum and the coccyx. These are at the bottom of the spine and extend into the pelvic area.

Within the top three regions of the spine, the vertebrae are all assigned numbers. So when there is a misalignment in a particular vertebra, the chiropractor may explain to the patient that there is a subluxation caused by the misalignment of the C4 vertebra. This would mean the 4th vertebra from the top, or the 4th vertebra in the cervical spine, is misaligned.

A patient who has a blockage or misalignment in the C4 vertebra could actually be seeing the doctor about their hay fever and not necessarily back pain. That is because the nerves that extend from the C4 vertebra are responsible for messages sent to the nose, lips, mouth, eustachian tube, and mucous membranes. Often a misalignment here manifests itself as hay fever, postnasal drip, adenoid infections, and other upper respiratory symptoms. There can even be problems with hearing by a misalignment of the C4 vertebra.

Every nerve that extends from the spinal column is responsible for an organ, function, or performance of some part of the body. This includes the obvious organs such as the sensory capabilities of touch, which goes literally to every part of the body. A complete body map shows this radial effect. If you were to envision an outline of the body and create lines from the center where the spine would be located, drawn out to each extremity, then you can see how the nerves and protective vertebrae are assigned to those areas within the body. You can also see clearly, then, how if the vertebra meant to protect the nerve gets pushed out of place, even slightly, how that can have an impact on the nerve signals that go out from that region of the spine.

This idea of the vertebrae being labeled and the corresponding nerves reaching out to all areas of the body is not exclusive to chiropractic. The medical field also recognizes the anatomy and what it means to have something out of alignment. Where mainstream medicine and chiropractic differ, is in the way it is treated and in recognizing the full impact of the misalignment.

HOW THE SPINE MOVES

The spine is able to bend and move and return to its "s"-like shape without incident or injury because of some of the soft tissue that works with the bony vertebrae. There are two types of soft tissue that are important in helping the spinal column protect the large central nerve, the spinal cord.

An inter-vertebral disk can be found between each vertebra. This disk helps absorb shock as the spine bends and twists during normal movement and activity. It also protects the vertebrae and spine from excessive shock. You don't think about that as you bend down to pick up a toy off the floor, because everything is in its proper place. You can even bend and twist to one side to grasp the toy that slid under the chair. However, if you were to have a deterioration of that disk or if it were to have slipped out of place even a little, there could be a grinding of the bone and a pinching of a nerve, and you would feel pain.

This type of back injury or painful condition is probably the number one reason people visit a chiropractor. Luckily, there are so many more health reasons that keep them returning to the chiropractor to maintain their overall health.

The second type of tissue is the facet joint. This allows for limited movement of the spine. The facet joints regulate movement so that routine movements are restricted to the point that they will not injure the spinal cord. The body, with its innate ability to heal, was created in a way that protects the most vital organs. The ribs protect the heart and lungs. The skull protects the brain. Then there is the spinal column to protect the spinal cord.

MISALIGNED VERTEBRAE

Every nerve in the body that radiates from the spinal cord supplies important information to the area of the body for which it is responsible. The example of the C4 vertebra being out of alignment is just one of literally hundreds of slight misalignments that can cause subluxation, that interference with the nerve signal, and result in some kind of ailment.

In the medical world, a patient visiting the doctor for indigestion or heartburn will almost immediately be prescribed some kind of antacid to ease those uncomfortable symptoms. For some people, this kind of quick fix may be okay for a while. After all, we all want to get rid of painful discomfort as quickly as possible. The problem with this treatment is that it doesn't cure the problem. It hardly even addresses the problem and certainly neglects the real cause of the problem. How can the body ever hope to heal itself if medications are momentarily quieting the symptoms?

Symptoms are there for a reason. The body, in its wisdom, has to let the brain know something isn't right. If we just quiet that inner voice with a medication, it's like telling someone to stop talking when they see you are about to get hit by a car. They are trying to give you an important message, but if you ignore it long enough, you will eventually have to deal with a much bigger problem.

When there is a symptom related to the stomach, it can often be traced back to the T6 vertebra. It is from this area that stomach problems and the body's ability to correct them transmit. The nerves in the T6 region could be experiencing some kind of interference. Removing that blockage through an adjustment of the spine will open up the lines of communication to the stomach and allow the problems in that region to be corrected naturally.

This simplified lesson on the anatomy of the spine is meant to illustrate the complex nature of the spinal column and the central nervous system. It is not quite as simple as explained here. There are so many minor misalignments that can impact one region of the body. Likewise, there are many different ways in which symptoms manifest themselves that it isn't always easy to pinpoint just what the real problem is. Back pain can often originate in the stomach and vice versa. Headaches can be the symptom for so many other ailments that may start out in a completely different area of the body. The complexities of this whole system is what chiropractors study for years so that they can perform the right diagnostic tests and begin the correct treatment for any specific ailment.

"DRUGS ARE NOT ALWAYS NECESSARY. BELIEF IN RECOVERY IS."

~NORMAN COUSINS

MANAGED CONDITIONS AND ILLNESSES

~8~

When most people think of a chiropractor, they tend to think of a doctor who manages and treats neck and back pain. Some might have a bit of a broader understanding of the science of chiropractic and know that chiropractors in fact handle most conditions associated with the musculoskeletal system and the nervous system. What many people don't yet know is that chiropractic deals with every system in the body. It can potentially help with any and every condition a person may have, and especially with the prevention of most illness and disease.

Since every organ and cell within the body is impacted by the central nervous system, it would make sense that any problems with the nervous system would lead to problems with the organ's function. This leads to illness and disease in the worst cases and a general feeling of malaise in the simplest cases.

Chiropractic cares for the nervous system by caring for the spine. The spine is the core of the nervous system and the protector of the spinal cord and each nerve. It can also act as the enemy to the nervous system in a sense when it's protective vertebrae that allow for movement and flexibility, become misaligned, and hinder the function of the nervous system. This is a condition in chiropractic that is referred to as subluxation.

A study conducted in Sweden by 87 different chiropractors sought to determine how patients responded to routine chiropractic care in ways other than benefits directly related to the musculoskeletal system. Twenty consecutive visits from patients for any reason were monitored. A total of 1,504 patients completed

[68]

questionnaires explaining where they noticed improvements in their symptoms for other conditions after receiving chiropractic treatment. Here are the amazing results:

No. of Patients	Positive Improvements in Non-Musculoskeletal Symptoms
98	Easier to breathe
92	Improved digestive function
49	Clearer/better/sharper vision
34	Improved circulation
10	Less ringing in the ears
8	Acne/eczema better
7	Dysmenorrhea better
6	Asthma/allergies better

STRESS

Emotional stress affects both men and women in different ways and the types of stress on a woman's system will result in different conditions. Many people will get headaches, suffer from insomnia, or develop digestive problems when the stresses of daily life go unchecked.

One example is that stress releases hormones which impact women, specifically by creating an imbalance in their overall endocrine system. Since the nervous system is the system that can regulate and bring back equilibrium to all other systems, it makes sense that chiropractic care can free up the nervous system to do its job.

There are many lifestyle changes that can be incorporated into everyone's routine. These not only include good eating habits and exercise, but ways to mentally reduce stress.

FIBROMYALGIA SYNDROME (FMS)

Fibromyalgia Syndrome (FMS) is a relatively unusual condition. For those it affects, however, it is an all consuming way of life compounded when it is not properly managed. Those who suffer from FMS, are so restricted in the everyday activities of life due to tenderness in the joints that they are ultimately controlled by the condition.

FMS is a chronic condition marked by tenderness and pain in many different points throughout the body. It is believed through extensive research that the root of the problem is either neurochemical, peripheral, or in the soft tissues. There are also hormonal imbalances found in patients with FMS that seem to have a connection, which makes sense when you understand that the nervous system and endocrine system, which encompass all of the hormones, are closely interconnected. In chiropractic we view and understand all systems to be connected to the nervous system, so it is understandable that chiropractic can help those with FMS.

Chiropractic has been extremely effective in helping those who suffer from FMS. The relief from pain that patients with FMS get is from the adjustments and procedures that get the nerves, joints, and muscles into optimal working order. Because those with FMS also suffer tenderness in all of the nodules, chiropractic care can help decrease the sensitivity to pain by helping the body properly metabolize waste and eliminate toxins.

There are lifestyle changes that go hand in hand with chiropractic to help relieve the pain of FMS. Dietary changes that include adequate amounts of magnesium help the patient to maintain proper pH balance. This allows better nerve transmission to the other nerves and muscles.

Keeping a routine schedule that includes plenty of exercise and sleep also helps alleviate FMS symptoms. Exercise, 20-30 minutes per day, done in the late afternoon or evening is most effective and promotes good sleep -- another way to battle FMS symptoms. Doing exercises in a swimming pool are great because there is not pressure or weight put on sensitive muscles.

"A MIRACLE DRUG IS ANY DRUG THAT WILL DO WHAT THE LABEL SAYS IT WILL DO."

~ERIC HODGINS

COPING WITH PERSONAL INJURIES

~9~

Personal injury is one of the most common reasons for first time visits to the chiropractor. It is also one that just about every insurance company will recognize as a necessary reason for being seen by a chiropractor. To start this chapter, let's just look at a quick definition of what "personal injury" really entails.

Personal injury ads appear on the television all the time. You've seen them. There is a lawyer swearing to get you everything you deserve because you have been injured by someone else's negligence. In reality, personal injury is not just an injury caused by another person, but any injury to your person.

Some of the more common types of injuries we get are the results of car accidents, sports injuries, those on the construction site or other work related injuries, or injuries from slightly overzealous "weekend warriors." These can include slips and falls, muscle strains and pulls, and even broken bones from working in the yard or around the house. Injury can occur from lifting and moving furniture, or even playing too hard with the kids. They are injuries from which the person usually makes a full recovery, but not without some aches and pains to go along with them. The injured person is usually better with a little first aid and some time to heal.

Let's take a closer look at each type of personal injury for which chiropractic can help.

AUTOMOBILE ACCIDENTS

Personal injury accounts for over 11,000 disabling injuries every hour of the entire year! It also seems as if personal injuries are on the rise. In 1995, construction workers reported more than 350,000 injuries, which was a 4% increase from the previous year. That wasn't even a close second to the number of automobile-related injuries in 1995. That number reached 5.5 million according to the National Highway Traffic Safety Administration. And even with higher safety standards and highway laws, such as lower speed limits, car accidents still accounted for 3.4 million injuries in 1999.

The pain and problems associated with car accidents can be realized even several years later. One of the most common types of car accident related injuries is to the neck. Chronic neck pain was felt by 39.6% of people who were in rear-end motor vehicle crashes even 7 years after the accident occurred.

When it comes to automobile accidents, men and women are not created equally. Women are more vulnerable to injury and more likely to suffer long-term consequences from a car accident. There are several reasons for this. One is they are usually lighter and therefore get thrown a bit more upon collision. The placement of the shoulder strap of the seatbelt is usually higher up on shorter people and therefore does not brace the upper body as well during a crash.

Neck injuries are not the only problems associated with automobile accidents. Chronic pain and many varying symptoms are the norm. The pain is not always felt immediately, which is a common occurrence with these types of soft tissue injuries. It usually takes about 2 weeks to start feeling the effects of damage to the spine and to soft tissues. What is actually happening is the beginning of a degenerative process of the spine which ultimately causes nerve damage. The good news is that these types of injuries can be corrected and stop further, permanent damage. If left untreated, then the victim runs the risk of permanent scar tissue forming which can result in chronic pain.

MUSCLE PULLS & STRAINS

It takes a 6% strain to cause a muscle to pull. Sometimes these pulls can be felt, but often they are not until much later in the day or even the next morning. What you cannot feel is that within one hour of causing the excess strain on the muscle, there is a 70% decrease in nerve function. Fortunately, with these minor pulls the nerve does return to full function usually within a day or two.

With more severe muscle pulls or strains, those around 12%, the nerve is completely blocked after about one hour. This type of muscle pull has minimal recovery and permanent damage leaves the nerve blocked to a degree that it no longer sends along important messages that keep you healthy. Treating soft tissues such as the muscles and nerves for pressure and strain is important in keeping them healthy. This includes even those strains we don't feel as strongly. That is another reason why regular, routine chiropractic care is so important and not just when you can feel the impact of the injury.

To get a good idea of what nerve pressure can do, compare it to the amount of pressure a dime would put on the nerve. A dime's worth of pressure is able to block away 60% of the nerves function. This is undetectable by the way you feel, but causes the nerve's function to be reduced by more than one-half.

Chiropractic can do a great deal to speed up the healing process, especially when the injury involves the spine and neck. By realigning the spine, even the soft tissue – pulled muscles and torn ligaments – are able to heal more quickly and completely, by re-opening the subluxation or blockage of nerve signals that may have resulted from the injury.

WHIPLASH

Whiplash occurs when there is a sudden jerk due to a change in motion. Most often it is associated with car accidents, because crashes result in sudden stopping, and that impact suddenly stops the forward motion of the vehicle. There are other ways to get whiplash and some important ways to prevent it as well.

Rear end collisions in an automobile cause a type of whiplash knows as extension-acceleration whiplash. This is considered the type of whiplash that causes the most damage. It can lead to degenerative disc disease in several disc levels – a process which takes about 7 years following the injury. Being caught off guard or by surprise increases the impact of whiplash. It also makes the long term prognosis worse especially for those who do not receive proper treatment.

Another factor that can increase the injury of whiplash is head rotation. If at the exact moment of impact the head is turning there is greater damage to the foramen, or holes between the vertebrae. This is because with a turned head this hole is compressed. With a compressed foramen there is more torque and that means more damage to the facets, capsules, and ligaments.

A turned head during impact also means there is greater hyperextension or flexion. This further increases the strain on soft tissues. In a nutshell, a turning head during impact causes more injury, even if the force of the collision is less.

Millions of people experience whiplash injury, some without even realizing it. Of the entire population, only one percent will have chronic neck pain associated with whiplash. Constant, severe, and indefinite neck pain will be felt by 10 percent of patients with whiplash injury.

There are other symptoms as well that develop and manifest themselves as pain that are associated with whiplash injury. Twenty-five percent of people with whiplash injuries will have life-long symptoms. The reason the symptoms are so severe and lasting is that with whiplash there is injury to the intervertebral discs, zygapophyseal joints, and/or alar ligaments. These are injuries that cannot correct themselves, and left untreated become chronic.

Since just about everyone can experience whiplash at some point in their lives, how can you know if you have whiplash? Whiplash can be marked by several symptoms. Some of the more common symptoms of whiplash include:

- Neck pain and/or stiffness
- Pain in the shoulders or between shoulder blades
- Headache
- Back pain

[77]

- Numbness or tingling
- Dizziness or a feeling of being lightheaded
- Pain in the arms, legs, ankles, feet, wrists, hands, or face and jaw
- Memory loss or trouble concentrating
- Blurred or double vision

You can even get whiplash sitting in an unmoving car if someone hits it from behind or the side. Whiplash can occur when a bicycle hits the curb. It could even occur on some amusement park rides and not just on the bumper cars. It can happen anywhere directions in the motion of the ride suddenly change or come to a sudden stop. No matter how you get whiplash, it can be more than just a pain in the neck. Whiplash can tear ligaments in the neck and upper back. It can cause muscle strain, making turning the head extremely painful.

The faster you can get chiropractic care following such an injury the better. A careful check of your neck and spine will allow for corrections in misalignments to begin immediately and help restore pain-free motion more quickly.

In 1996, a retrospective study of patients with chronic whiplash syndrome indicated that 93% benefited from chiropractic treatment. Treatment included controlled mobilization as opposed to completely immobilizing the injured area. Controlled movement is able to spark a reaction in the nerves that actually decreases pain. Mobilization has proven more effective in treating musculoskeletal soft tissue injuries. This type of treatment gets people back into full activity quicker while not negatively impacting the long-term recuperation.

SLIPS & FALLS

Slips and falls is actually a technical term used in the commercial real estate injury. It refers to injuries that can occur on the premises of a business and often leaves the building owner or manager liable for any injury caused by a slip or fall on their property. They work diligently to prevent these types of personal injuries both for the sake of their tenants and visitors and to protect themselves against liability.

The injuries that come from slips and falls are often not noticeable on the outside. There could be some minor scrapes or bruises, but most often there is substantial injury that goes unnoticed for a period of time. It may be days later before the symptoms of some internal movement of the spine from "catching" yourself and jerking in a strange way as you fall could even show up.

It is important if you have fallen to be checked out from a chiropractic perspective. You may have covered the scrape with a bandage and gone on your way, just happy that not too many people actually saw you fall! The important part of caring for your spine after such a fall is to be sure that your vertebrae were not thrown out of alignment. In the long run, that could lead to far more serious health problems down the road.

SPORTS INJURIES

There are obvious injuries for which chiropractic is not the first course of action. For many people receiving a sports-related injury, often the first step is to ice the injured area to draw away the blood. This will help reduce swelling immediately. Broken bones must be X-rayed and the best time and place to do this is usually immediately and at the closest emergency room.

It is the long-term effects of a sports injury for which chiropractic care can offer the best long-term treatments and results. A chiropractor will generally take their own X-rays following a sports injury as well as reference the first X-rays taken following the injury. Depending on the type and location of the injury, treatments will vary.

One example of a common sports-related injury is twisted or sprained ankle. This happens to athletes of all ages and abilities. Now many people may think the chiropractor only comes in when there is a neck or back injury, but even healing in the ankle can be referenced back to an area in the spine and nerve signals that originate in the spinal cord. Again, the soft tissue is affected with a sprain.

By ensuring there is no subluxation in the vertebra corresponding to the legs, ankles and feet, the soft tissue will be restored to its optimal state as quickly as possible. It just makes sense when you really look at the process of spraining an ankle. Not just the ankle is affected. Chances are that in the process of twisting there could be falling. But even more significant is that when someone twists and turns and ankle, their entire torso centered with the spine also twists in an unnatural manner.

OTHER INJURIES

I don't know if people are generally just a little clumsy or if there is another reason why almost everyone at some point in their life gets injured doing every day things. It's easy to see and understand how it happens to children. They may be riding a bike for the first time and fall off. They may underestimate their abilities to jump down from a tree limb. They may just be moving too quickly that the development of their coordination has not yet caught up with their desire to go and do new things.

Whatever the reason, we all get injured in some way that at the very least causes pain and discomfort. At the worst, our personal injuries cause permanent changes in our abilities to do something we love.

Chiropractic's main objective is to open the body up to its full potential. That potential refers to its ability to heal itself and organize every system within itself through innate intelligence to do all for which it was designed. Another equally important objective is to allow people to live life to the fullest. That generally means as healthy and happy as possible. I have found that health does often equal happiness and that illness and disease can often depress both the body and the spirit.

When you experience an injury or illness for that matter, the body knows what to do to protect itself and the injured area. When there is an infection, the body increases its white blood cell count and produces a burning fever to rid the body as quickly as possible from the infection. When you put out that fire with a fever-reducing medicine, the uncomfortable symptom of fever is gone, but the infection is allowed to live on. These symptoms can also accompany an injury.

REDUCING INJURY

The best way to treat an injury is to avoid it. Here are some tips on lifting, working, and playing that will help reduce your incidents of injury. Then if you do get injured, be sure that part of your treatment is to visit the chiropractor to remove any subluxation which will allow the body to heal quickly and completely.

Lifting

- *Use your legs to lift heavy objects.* Squat and reach under the object, then stand so your legs take the brunt of the weight and not your back.

- *Get help.* Ask someone else to help you lift awkwardly shaped objects. Even if they are not overly heavy, trying to maneuver them can cause strain and injury.

- *Use moving disks.* There are Teflon® coated disks that can be placed under furniture that allows you to easily slide even very heavy pieces without lifting. One disk goes under each corner (remember to lift corners using your legs to hold the weight) and then the furniture can slide over wood, tile, or carpeted floors.

- *Use a cart to move heavy objects.*

- *Wear a specialized lifting* belt to hold stomach muscles supporting the back tightly in place.

[82]

Working around the House

- When completing any chore it is a good idea to not do any one movement or motion for too long of a period of time. The constant repetitive motion can cause injury. This includes raking, vacuuming, painting, gardening, etc.

- Don't sit or stand in one position for too long without changing position. If you are peeling large amounts of vegetables for canning or working at the computer you can be standing or sitting in the same position for too long.

- Vary your tasks for a given day. Do a little shoveling, then switch to walking or a sitting activity every hour or so.

Avoiding Injuries from Riding

- Always wear a helmet when riding a bicycle or motorcycle.

- Always wear a shoulder restraint seat belt in the car.

- Keep your seat belt on when flying in an airplane. You will be protected from unexpected turbulence.

[83]

Preparing Yourself to Workout or Play

- Warm up muscles gradually by starting out slowly when walking and running, then increase speed and intensity.

- Wear the proper shoes for any sports activity or walking.

- Stretch muscles following a workout while they are still warm.

- If you have been inactive, don't jump into a game you are not conditioned to play. Work yourself up gradually over weeks and months to that level of play.

Chiropractic vs. Physical Therapy

Often following an injury, a medical doctor will recommend physical therapy. I recommend it as well in conjunction with proper chiropractic care. There are some differences in the treatment provided by both and they can complement each other.

Normally, a physical therapist will do similar tests to that of a chiropractor in treating a patient recovering from an injury. Range of motion and pain sensitivity is tested along with muscular responses to certain stimuli. The physical therapist will then work with the patient to make movements to the body that will increase motion, flexibility, and overall functionality to the injured area. The chiropractor is involved in some of this but takes the process one step further. This extra step is extremely critical to a full and complete recovery if one is to be possible.

Chiropractic also looks at range of motion, flexibility, and restoration of the full function of the injured area. The extra step is in the area of the "full function." If, for example, there is an injury to one's shoulder, the physical therapist is looking at making it so the patient can move the arm and shoulder without pain. The chiropractor does as well. The next step that the chiropractor takes is to ensure there is nothing prohibiting that range of motion and the healing power of the body to restore the soft tissues that may have been injured.

Pain has an interesting way of showing up in a place other than where you are actually injured. A physical therapist and the medical field as a whole may be looking solely at where the pain is actually located. They may not be focusing completely or at all on the actual source of the pain. With full chiropractic care the entire nervous system is freed to begin real healing. In other words, a pain in the shoulder may actually be caused by a subluxation caused by a misaligned vertebra in the neck.

BACK PAIN

Chronic back and neck pain are some of the most common reasons for visiting the chiropractor. They are also a top reason many people visit their medical doctor. In fact, it is estimated that 4 out of 5 adults will experience back pain at some point in their lives and many suffer from chronic back pain. It is usually this latter group of people that seek long term care for the management of the pain.

The lower back could be referred to as the keystone of the body. It's what holds us upright as we walk and, as such an important part of our structure, it needs to be cared for properly.

There are also many, many environmental factors that can affect the wellness of the lower back. Our jobs, the way we lift, the style of shoes we wear, our sleep positions and mattress quality all impact our lower back. In fact, all these factors can form the lower back in such a unique way that no two people have exactly the same structural balance in their backs. Add to that our own genetic makeup and it is easy to see how our backs can get molded into different shapes – some good, and some not so well.

If you are carrying around extra weight, you are also forming your lower back into a shape that may not be conducive to good spinal health. This can compress bones and put pressure on the vertebrae, which can block good nerve signals from passing through the spine.

In a perfect world, everyone would be their ideal weight and have a job that supports a healthy spine. Fashion trends would put us all in low-heeled wide shoes, or better yet, let us go barefoot. Because we add these stresses to our spine, it is more important than ever to get regular chiropractic adjustments to correct minor shifts before they become major subluxations, those interferences with nerve signals.

[86]

Without the proper back care, one of the most common complaints is lower back pain. This can be in the form of sciatica, where pain radiates down the leg from the large sciatic nerve. It can also caused by injury or inflammation of the soft tissues between the vertebrae.

In treating different types of back pain, good medical doctors will do a great deal to determine the cause of the pain, but are usually very quick to prescribe pain medication to alleviate the symptoms while the process of elimination is completed. Patients are often so satisfied with the short-term absence of pain that comes from these strong medications, that they continue taking the pain killers and postpone or avoid all together further steps to determine the cause of the pain.

There are several problems with this type of treatment of back pain. One is that it is a short-term solution and often leaves the patient dependent on medication. Secondly, without addressing the source of the pain – by ignoring the symptoms the body is telling the brain -- you could be ignoring a more serious problem. Finally, most pain medications will become ineffective over time, making it necessary to take more and more in order to get the same results. This vicious cycle of either changing medications every few months or increasing the dosage can lead to problems with addiction.

TREATING CHRONIC BACK PAIN

There are three main stages to treating chronic back pain, and none has to include surgery. Before any long-term treatment can be effective, the

[87]

inflammation that is causing the pain must be reduced. As long as there is inflammation there will be pressure on the nerves and there will be pain. That is why this is the first stage in treating chronic back pain.

Two of the best, non-surgical methods of reducing inflammation without medication, is rest and ice. Resting for one to two weeks relieves strains that can keep the swelling inflamed. Icing also reduces inflammation by drawing the blood away from the injury.

Once the inflammation is gone, therapy to strengthen the rested muscles again and help prevent future injuries can begin. In this second stage, simple exercises are repeated for about two weeks (sometimes longer) until the movements can be made with greater ease and without pain.

The third stage is the life-long changes in lifestyle that will let you carry on with life free from back pain. It may mean changing habits such as sitting in one position for too long of a period of time or holding the telephone to your ear with one shoulder so both hands are free to cook. It may mean if you drive for long distances that you use a pillow to alter the way you sit to improve your posture.

All of these little habits many people have can be adding each day to future or current back pain. Little changes made for a lifetime can lead to a lifetime of freedom from back and neck pain without surgery or drugs.

In chiropractic, medication is not part of the back pain solution. Getting to the root of the problem is. A study conducted on chronic lower back pain sought to determine whether chiropractic or other medical treatment was more effective in treating lower back pain. The findings may surprise you.

The outcome was that both were effective in treating the pain just about equally. Disability from the back pain was also treated about as well with chiropractic and medical treatment. The biggest differences reported by patients were in the level of care they received and their overall satisfaction with the process. Remember that the medical treatment included medication that can be costly and addictive. The chiropractic treatment did not.

Some of the other significant findings from the study were:

- *No leg pain was found with the lower back pain in 41% of patients who saw a chiropractor compared with 27% of medical patients who said there was no leg pain.*

- *73% of chiropractic patients were satisfied with* the amount of information given them *vs. 40% of medical patients.*

- *82% of chiropractic patients left feeling they knew how to better care for their back vs. 51% of medical patients.*

- *74% of chiropractic patients were confident their treatment for lower back pain was working vs. 36% of medical patients.*

- *83% of chiropractic patients would choose a doctor of chiropractic again for treatment vs. 61% of medical patients would choose a medical doctor again for the same treatment of lower back pain.*

THE SLIPPED DISC

A slipped or herniated disc is a condition in which a disc, the soft tissue of cartilage in between the vertebrae, has slipped out of place slightly causing swelling or bulging. Even minor swelling can cause pressure on the nerves corresponding to that disc and pain in the area supplied by that nerve. This is one reason why leg, neck, or shoulder pain will occur when there is a problem within in the spinal region.

There are many misconceptions with chiropractic care for a slipped disc. You may have heard that when there is a chiropractic adjustment the doctor is "popping" a disc into place. This idea may sound painful and it could be if it were really what was happening!

When a chiropractor works to correct disc problems it is with gentle pressure and only after proper diagnostic testing. The sound of "popping" that you may have heard about is actually gases being released from the tissue. If there is any "pain" experienced, it is in the form of a minor, very short-lived discomfort.

Manipulative treatment for a slipped disc occurs over a period of time with several applications of light pressure and movement. It cannot be fixed with one quick "pop." There are also cases where manipulation is not the appropriate

[90]

course of action and where in the end, a spinal surgeon may need to be consulted. These are only the very extreme and rare situations.

Some of the diagnostic techniques that the chiropractor uses in determining the right treatment for a slipped disc are the X-ray, CAT scan, and the MRI. An X-ray focuses in on the skeletal system, by passing the skin and soft tissue. It is one of the most common ways to take a good picture of bones.

A CAT or Computerized Axial Tomography scan uses many X-rays projected at different angles to review various layers of tissue. It can view the tissue in such small increments that any type of lesion or abnormality in the tissue is easily seen. This is often the way cancerous tissues in the very early stages are detected.

Finally, the most sensitive image comes from the MRI or Magnetic Resonance Imaging. No radiation is used with the MRI and it is able to focus in directly on thin slices or layers of tissue in even smaller increments than the CAT scan. There is virtually nothing that cannot be detected in the soft tissues of the discs and nerves through the keen images of the MRI

All chiropractors are trained in interpreting the images seen from these diagnostic tools. Many of the tests can even be performed in the office. On occasion, X-rays are done at a local medical facility. Because of the extreme specialization of the MRI machinery, those tests are performed by specialists at a local medical center and then the films become part of the chiropractor's records.

One test specific to chiropractic in determining areas of disc problems is palpation or touch. This is done while the patient is performing certain movements and also without movement. Chiropractors will palpate muscles in a similar fashion to determine if there are areas of weakness. The results of these tests along with X-rays, CAT scans, or MRIs, will dictate the course of treatment.

The process of easing a slipped disc back into place and normal function is accompanied by constant updating of information received directly from the patient. Throughout the process the patient is asked about pain levels, mobility, and how they are feeling in general. If the pain lessens and mobility increases, then follow up treatments are administered to keep progressing in the right direction throughout the healing process.

SCIATICA

Sciatica is a term used by the lay person in a very general sense for just about any pain in the upper gluteus area that then causes radial pain down the legs. It is actually a little more complicated than that, and for neurologists and doctors of chiropractic, there are many specific conditions that can be lumped into the general category of sciatica. Each would have slightly different symptoms and require different courses of action.

This broad definition of sciatica is referring to conditions related to the sciatic nerve. The sciatic nerve is the largest nerve in the body. It runs from the lumbar spine through the sacrum at the bottom of the spine and is responsible for feeling in all parts of the legs, knees, ankles, and feet. The sciatic nerve is about ¾

[92]

inch in diameter and then branches off at the pelvis. Any inflammation or injury to the sciatic nerve is therefore referred to as sciatica.

Sciatica is a common condition but can leave the patient with a great deal of lower back and leg pain. It makes everyday activities -- including sitting, walking, and even standing -- difficult and painful. With more extreme swelling there can even be a loss of reflexes and muscle strength in the legs.

The good news about sciatica, if there can be anything good about leg pain, is that it is effectively treated without surgery or the use of steroids to reduce the inflammation. Chiropractic adjustments, to release some of the pressure from swelling of the nerve and to allow uninterrupted nerve signals to flow, make for quick and complete recovery.

Sciatica is also managed well with physical therapy that can be taught and monitored by the chiropractor. Most of the therapy can be done at home with simple activities after the initial phases of treatment. After a period of allowing the muscles to rest, short periods of walking and stretching can begin, gradually working up to normal activity levels. In rare cases, surgery may be required to relieve pressure from swelling, or repair damage or degeneration to the disc associated with the sciatica.

SCOLIOSIS

Scoliosis is often associated with teenage girls as described in "coming of age" novels. The girls are described as having to wear hideous braces on their backs and face the humiliation of adolescence with one more obstacle. It is true that childhood scoliosis is often diagnosed in the pre-teen years and is more common in girls. However, it can go unnoticed until adulthood and affect boys too.

It is "Idiopathic" scoliosis that is most associated with childhood, although it may not show up until much later in life. It is a hereditary condition or disease and cannot be prevented, but treated before it worsens.

Scoliosis in the literal definition means curvature. It is an "s" or "c" curve to the spine that goes from side to side. The spine naturally curves from front to back in a slight "s" shape. The curvature from side to side is measured in degrees as the curves are detected by X-ray, but it can often be detected by a child's pediatrician or chiropractor. Sometimes a noticeable unevenness in the shoulders or hips is the first tell-tale sign.

Scoliosis is best treated while the child is still growing. During the teen years, when there are huge growth spurts, a brace can be worn to correct the shape of the spine. This type of non-surgical treatment is the least invasive and is extremely effective. There are also exercises that can be done to keep muscles stronger and help hold the spine into the proper position. These exercises also act as therapy for any pain associated with the disease. Frequent spinal adjustments to correct the growth pattern of the spine work in conjunction with physical therapies. As a last resort, spinal surgery may be required.

CARPAL TUNNEL SYNDROME

Carpal Tunnel Syndrome (CTS) is one of three common repetitive stress injuries. The others are trigger finger and nerve spasms. The term repetitive stress injury simply means that the condition is caused by doing something over and over again for a period of months or sometimes years, and in a way that puts stress on a part of the body.

Repetitive stress injuries may have been around since the cave men rubbed sticks together repeatedly, but it was only given the name of Carpal Tunnel Syndrome in the last 20 or so years. This is when computers became widely used in homes and offices. Extended periods of time at the computer day in and day out are still one of the leading occupational hazards resulting in CTS. Up until this point, primarily grocery store clerks (pre-bar code era) and accountants used the repetitive finger motions enough to cause CTS.

In the case of Carpal Tunnel Syndrome, the stress is placed on the carpel tunnel. This small canal inside the wrist is actually made up of three parts: the median nerve; nine flexor tendons; and blood vessels. When someone is diagnosed with Carpel Tunnel Syndrome there is some sort of compression of the median nerve. This can reveal itself with several symptoms. Most common are numbness and tingling in the wrist and hand, weakness and/or clumsiness in the hands, neck tension, swelling, and sometimes night pain.

Traditionally, medical doctors have placed their focus in dealing with carpel tunnel syndrome on the wrist and hands themselves. After all, this is where you feel most of the pain. What they don't seem to focus on is the fact that

[95]

leading to the carpel tunnel is the median nerve. This pain's journey actually begins in the neck, goes under the collar bone, and on to the wrist and hand through the carpal tunnel.

The most common course of action is to prescribe anti-inflammatory and pain killing drugs known as NSAIDS. These are the non-steroidal type of drugs that come with some serious side effects and offer only a temporary relief from pain. They do nothing to treat the cause of CTS. In the United States alone, there are approximately 16,000 deaths per year from the misuse of NSAIDS. This is the Advil and Aleve type medications and includes different forms of aspirin. Extensive use of these drugs causes bleeding within the lining of the stomach and intestines, which can lead to death.

To treat Carpal Tunnel Syndrome in a lasting manner and without surgery, you must find out where the median nerve is being compressed. That could be anywhere from the neck down to the hand. There are several ways in which the median nerve can become compressed. They include:

- *Misaligned bones in the neck*
- *Tight neck muscles and/or forearm muscles*
- *Shoulder dysfunction*
- *Inflamed tendons*

These are caused by:

- *Poor posture*
- *Repetitive movements*

[96]

- *Rapid finger movements*

- *Improper movements*

- *Poor ergonomics*

- *Slips or falls*

- *Sleeping on your stomach with your hands underneath*

- *Certain sports and hobbies such as bowling, racquetball, and motorcycling*

There are other causes of Carpal Tunnel Syndrome, but they are extremely rare. Some systemic diseases where water in retained, such as diabetes, can cause compression on the median nerve. Pregnancies, use of birth control pills, and high salt diets have all occasionally caused CTS.

The chiropractic approach to treating Carpel Tunnel Syndrome is completely different from a medical doctor's point of view. Chiropractors do not focus on the wrist or hand, but the cause of compression in the median nerve. To diagnose this, a complete evaluation of the patient's lifestyle, along with a surface postural exam, will give the chiropractor a good picture of the source of compression.

The surface postural exam is a computerized test that measures how hard the spinal muscles are pulling on each the left and right sides of the body. It is used to evaluate how well balanced the muscular system is. (There is that word "balanced" again used with chiropractic!) If there are imbalances in the muscles in the neck, it is a good indication that the median nerve is compressed and is the primary cause of the Carpel Tunnel Syndrome.

Testing for CTS

Another test you can use at home involves holding your hands in a position where the backs are pressed together with the fingers pointing down and the elbows out to the side. The wrists should be bent at a 90 degree angle. If this position is uncomfortable or if after one minute there is numbness or pain, you may have Carpal Tunnel Syndrome. To be sure, the surface postural exam or an electromyography (EMG) exam must be implemented. The EMG sends a small electrical current through the wrist which should travel at a rate of 13 meters per second. If it is slower, then it is likely that there is nerve damage or compression.

Preventing & Treating CTS

Therapies to treat Carpal Tunnel Syndrome include an alignment of specific neck vertebra and relieving tension in the muscles in the neck. It does not include drugs or surgery.

There are nutritional precautions that you can take to ensure a healthy median nerve and tissues surrounding the carpal tunnel. For example, Coenzyme Q10 helps improve tissue oxygenation. B complex vitamins support choline and inositol that enhance nerve function. B6 has diuretic properties that can relieve pressure on the nerve caused by fluid retention. Finally, zinc enhances general healing.

In addition to the minerals, there are herbs that support flexibility and reduce inflammation. Some good herbs are Aloe Vera and Marshmallow root. To relieve muscle spasms and pain, Skullcap is a good herb.

Everyday dietary choices can also help prevent Carpal Tunnel Syndrome. You should avoid high sodium foods, especially processed foods, because they will cause you to retain fluids. Likewise, drinking plenty of water will help flush out excess fluids.

To prevent joints from swelling and possibly putting pressure on the median nerve, avoid foods that contain large amounts of oxalic acid. This means asparagus, eggs, fish, and any vegetables in the cabbage family, which should be eaten sparingly.

You can take measures to prevent Carpal Tunnel Syndrome each day by being conscious of your positions and varying movements. Here are some guidelines:

- *Hold on to objects with the entire hand and not just gripping with the fingers. An example is the plastic grocery bags. Don't ever just hook the heavy bags on your fingers; use the whole hand to support the weight.*

- *Position yourself at the computer with the monitor just below your line of vision. Make sure the entire forearm is supported so that wrists are not bent up or down while typing. You can add a wrist pad to the bottom of the keyboard to keep wrists straight.*

[99]

- *Stop, rest, change position, and shake wrists periodically. Try to do repetitive typing jobs in short bursts with good, long breaks in between.*

- *Restore the circulation to your wrists and stretch and exercise them often by gently rotating them for about 2 minutes.*

"WHEN THE HEAD ACHES, ALL THE BODY IS THE WORSE."

~ENGLISH PROVERB

HEADACHES: SIGN OR SYMPTOM?

~10~

Headaches deserve a section all of their own. This is because headaches are probably one of the most common reasons for which someone goes to their doctor or chiropractor for pain relief. In the year 2000, it is estimated that 45 million Americans with headaches went to their doctor, adding up to 50 million office visits. This resulted in 157 million missed days of work and an expenditure of $2 billion for just over-the-counter pain medications.

When someone goes to the doctor with a headache, often the questioning revolves around eyesight, sinuses, and migraines. The cure is usually a pain medication that gives temporary relief, but does little to solve the core problem.

The pain medications most often prescribed also have an addictive quality that not only "hooks" the patient, but makes it so that more and more of the medicine is required to relieve the pain. The patient builds up a tolerance for the drug to the point that even the highest doses are ineffective in relieving the pain.

There are a few things you should keep in mind when you take these pain relievers. Most important of all is: A HEADACHE IS NOT AN ILLNESS – IT IS A SYMPTOM!

You are only temporarily treating a symptom when you take a pain reliever, not getting to the root of the problem. If you take medication to get rid of the pain, you are only masking the pain, but not treating the source of the pain.

Without finding and treating the reason for the headache, it is bound to return again and again, beginning a cycle that will be difficult to break.

Rebound Headaches are the result of frequently taking pain medications for headaches. If you take pain relievers more than twice a week for a headache, you may actually be getting headaches more often as your body begins to rely on the pain medication.

Once you start on the rebound cycle, it can be very difficult to break out of it. Some headache sufferers soon find themselves taking medication daily to keep headaches at bay. After a while, they find themselves taking medication as if they were snacking on candy.

Taking pain medications too often leads to a variety of problems, including:

- *Increased dependence on pain relievers*
- *Increased tolerance on pain medications so that you must take higher and higher dosages as time goes on*

- *Irritation of the stomach and intestines with repeated use, leading to side effects such as ulcers and gastrointestinal bleeding*

That's why it is so important to get past masking the pain and move on to getting to the source and stopping the headache before it starts.

[103]

Coping with Headaches

Many people have come to simply live with their headaches and cope. This is because pain medication up to this point has only offered them a short-term bandage to cover up the symptoms to let them get on with their work and their lives, if even only for a few hours.

There are several other reasons why headaches need to be dealt with head on, so to speak. Headaches often do the following:

- Cause relationships to suffer because of cancelled plans, increased tension, irritability. All of the misery that recurring pain triggers can have a lasting effect on your loved ones.
- Cause you to have to withdraw into your room to "sleep it off."
- Short-change yourself and your family from time together.

Headache Classifications

To take the next step in headache treatment you have to understand the source of the headache. Only then can the forces within the body be awakened. Only then can healing begin and the big cover-up end.

Although it is not known exactly what causes headaches, healthcare professionals do know that there are certain triggers to different kinds of headaches. Theoretically then, by avoiding these triggers you can avoid the headache.

One of the biggest obstacles to figuring out the exact type of headache and what triggers it is that there are so many different types of headaches. For this reason, back in 1988 the International Headache Society (IHS) came up with a way to classify headaches based on symptoms, frequency, and research by the health community. The list was updated in 2004 to place headaches into one of 15 different categories listed here as published by IHS:

1. *Migraine*

2. *Tension-type headache*

3. *Cluster headaches and other trigeminal autonomic cephalalgias*

4. *Cervicogenic headaches*

5. *Other primary headaches*

6. *Headache associated with head trauma*

7. *Headaches associated with vascular disorders*

8. *Headaches associated with nonvascular intracranial disorder*

9. *Headache associated with substances or their withdrawal*

10. *Headache associated with infection*

11. *Headache attributed to disorder of homeostasis*

12. *Headache or facial pain attributed to disorder of cranium, neck, eyes, ears, nose, sinuses, teeth, mouth, or other facial or cranial structures*

13. *Headache attributed to psychiatric disorder*

14. *Cranial neuralgias and central causes of facial pain*

15. *Other headaches, cranial neuralgia, central or primary facial pain*

This classification system has become the standard by which most headaches are diagnosed. It is used by physicians and chiropractors alike.

[105]

Drawing from the specific classifications, there are different categories of headache that are further classified as either primary or secondary. Most, 90%, of all headaches are primary in nature, meaning they are not part of another medical condition. These primary headaches are all the result of some kind of upset in the neurotransmitters of the brain – a primary condition addressed by chiropractic.

Secondary headaches, on the other hand, include what is known as rebound headaches. This occurs when too much aspirin or other analgesic medications are used. So by taking this type of medication in excess, research has found that you are actually causing more headaches.

Primary headaches top the classification list for the most common types of headaches, the three most common types being Migraine, Tension, and Cluster headaches.

MIGRAINE HEADACHES

Migraines are some of the most severe forms of headaches. Approximately 13% or 28 million adults get migraine headaches. These throbbing headaches usually occur on one side of the head or the other and last from between 4 and 72 hours, hitting at various, unpredictable times. Other symptoms that accompany a migraine headache include sensitivity to light and noise, and sometimes odors that induce nausea or vomiting.

Other symptoms of a migraine headache may include:

[106]

- A pre-headache phase where sensory perceptions seem enhanced. Colors seem brighter, a feeling of "butterflies in the stomach," and a light, disoriented feeling may wash over you.
- An "aura" will begin before the headache strikes as visual disturbance such as flashing, flickering lights in one corner of your field of vision.

There are factors known to contribute to the onset and severity of a migraine headache. Unfortunately, they are also some people's most favorite indulgences. Migraines may be triggered by caffeine, alcohol, and cigarette smoke. Even if you don't drink coffee, smoke, or partake of alcoholic beverages, you can set off a migraine in other ways. These include chocolate, the common preservative MSG, some prescription medications, or even by smelling gasoline or different perfumes.

Other environmental factors that can lead to a migraine are the weather changes, bright lights, and loud noises. You can get migraines by becoming fatigued or not dealing with emotional stress.

There are some health conditions that can contribute to migraines. Often dealing with the other health problems will eliminate the migraine or prevent one from happening if you are prone to migraine headaches. Some of the more common ailments that lead to migraines are urinary tract infections, stomach trouble, or dysmenorrhea.

Migraines originate in arteries and veins in the brain and around the skull. Most susceptible are the cranial nerves and the covering to the brain known as the dura mater. They become inflamed and even infected, causing pain. Also pain can come from a compression or other irritations to the vessels.

Migraine headaches occur in a variety of forms, including classic migraines, common migraines and cluster migraines. Each type of migraine will respond to different types of treatment, and each person responds differently to chiropractic treatment. Migraine therapy must be custom tailored to the individual after a careful analysis and consultation with your chiropractor.

Chiropractic is very well equipped to deal with the root source of pain associated with a migraine headache. Because chiropractic deals with the nerves in the entire body, a problem with the cranial nerves and nerves that supply the blood vessels to the brain and head, it can effectively remove disturbances to these areas through spinal manipulation.

TENSION HEADACHES

Tension headaches are the most common type of headache experienced and almost all adults will experience at least one tension headache at one time or another.

The symptoms of a tension headache include:

- *A steady ache that usually feels like pressure or tightening around the skull*
- *Is usually felt on both sides of the head*

[108]

- *Is sometimes the result of eye strain, such as working on a computer or reading for long periods*
- *Can be stress related*
- *Does not usually have other symptoms like nausea*
- *Is sometimes accompanied by tightness or pain in the neck and/or shoulders*

Chiropractic soft tissue therapy is very effective in treating tension headaches.

Tension headaches are probably on the lower part of the pain scale, but can lead to pain in places other than the head. Back and neck pain are commonly associated with tension headaches as well. The tension headache is one of the most common types of headaches and starts at the base of the skull, but can radiate through the whole head.

Much of what attributes to a tension headache is stress. This kind of emotional or physical stress leads to muscle tension. Muscle tension in the neck and back can then lead to misalignments as tight muscles pull on the vertebrae.

CLUSTER HEADACHES

Cluster headaches are named as such because of the way they start behind the eyes and go out in cyclical patterns. These headaches come on suddenly and are quite severe on the pain scale. They are not the most common primary headaches, but do still attack approximately 1 million Americans. More than 90 percent of cluster headache sufferers are male.

[109]

Cluster headaches are treated by the medical profession much like other types of headaches, only with different types of drug therapies. Chiropractic addresses the root cause of the cluster headache and the nerve interference that corresponds to this headache pattern.

CERVICOGENIC HEADACHES

Cervicogenic headaches are a relatively recent classification of headache only now being given real attention by the medical community. Cervicogenic headaches differ from tension headaches in one very important aspect – abnormalities in the cervical area contribute to these headaches. Because they are musculoskeletal in origin, they will require different treatment than a standard tension headache.

The symptoms of a Cervicogenic headache include:

- *Non-throbbing pain that often begins in the neck and can fluctuate in severity over time*
- *Pain that can increase or be aggravated by neck movement*
- *Restricted range of movement in the neck*
- *Pain is often on one side of the head, and does not migrate or shift to the other side*
- *Often occurs after stress to the neck, such as a minor accident or twisting and turning such as when doing work like wallpapering or sitting in front of a computer for long stretches*

While Cervicogenic headaches respond well to soft tissue therapy, the best treatment is most often a combination of soft tissue therapy and spinal manipulation. Cervicogenic headaches are one of the most often mis-diagnosed type of headaches by the medical mainstream, as they are a relatively new classification of headache and are related closely to the misalignment of the seven cervical vertebrae in the neck.

OTHER CAUSES OF HEADACHE

There are other causes of headaches that cannot necessarily be classified as a specific type of headache. The everyday occurrences that can bring on a headache can be determined by a chiropractic exam.

Simple Muscle Tension

Muscle tension can be caused by anything from eye strain to sitting in one position for too long a period of time. As your body becomes fatigued, the muscles tighten up in an effort to maintain proper alignment and this tightening can lead to real pain.

Subluxation

A subluxation occurs when a group of vertebrae is out of alignment, leading to a cascade of other problems. When vertebrae are out of alignment, the ligaments connecting them contract around these areas, adapting to the abnormal posture.

[111]

Muscles will then begin to spasm in an attempt to prevent further misalignment and to compensate for the current misalignment or misalignments. This causes pain which often is "referred" to the skull and reveals itself as a headache. In advanced cases, the discs between the vertebrae can degenerate, causing additional pain.

Subluxation also results in pinching of the nerves and blood vessels in the area around the vertebrae. This pressure on the nerve endings causes pain, and constriction of blood vessels and reduces the amount of blood and oxygen to the brain, which can also lead to headache pain. This is often the case with severe headaches such as migraines.

TREATING HEADACHES WITH CHIROPRACTIC

If you have frequent headaches, regardless of whether they are tension headaches, Cervicogenic, or migraines, you may also be suffering from rebound headaches. There are several warning signs that indicate rebound headaches:

- *Headaches are daily or more than two or three times a week*
- *There is no medical reason for your headaches*
- *You often wake up with a headache*
- *The headache often returns about the time your pain medication begins to "wear off." (4-5 hours for something like Tylenol, 8-12 hours for Aleve)*
- *Headaches are often triggered by minor exertion or mental concentration*
- *You have been increasing your dosage of pain medications to find relief*
- *The headaches have become closer together over time*

[112]

If you are experiencing rebound headaches, you should consider just how serious they can be. Taking pain medications several times a week not only masks the actual cause of your headaches, it will, over time, begin to interfere with your body's own ability to handle pain.

The human body produces endorphins which alleviate pain, but the daily use of painkillers interferes with this natural process, making you more dependent on medications over time. This leads to the rebound effect that is so frustrating. The only way to stop this cycle is to stop taking the daily or almost daily doses of pain medication so that your body can begin handling the pain on its own again. This can be difficult in the first week or so, but with proper chiropractic care, you can get rid of the primary headaches so that the rebound headaches won't continue to be an issue!

Chiropractors are able to perform some simple tests and examinations to determine more specifically the cause of a headache. These tests, along with questions about your lifestyle, help the chiropractor take a look at every facet of your life in order to understand how different situations or factors interact in your life to trigger recurring headaches.

The tests and procedures include but are not limited to:

- *A physical examination including blood tests, vital signs, reflexes and several other tests as well as orthopedic and range of motion tests and specific orthopedic and neurological exams, if needed*

[113]

- *X-rays may be taken of the bones, discs, and soft tissues of the neck area in order to evaluate the condition of the structures supporting the neck and head.*

- *Static Posture-Pro Testing, which is a new form of imaging that determines abnormal functioning of the muscles that support the head.*

There is vital balance the body strives to maintain between the muscular system, the skeletal system, and the central nervous system. When one of these systems is disturbed, damaged, or out of balance it will inevitably effect the others. Discussing and evaluating all of these with your chiropractor will help ensure that your treatment addresses all of the various causes of headache pain you may have.

After an initial consultation to determine the type of headaches you are suffering from (and there could be more than one!), a chiropractor will develop an individualized program developed specifically for you that may include several different types of treatment. These courses of treatment will depend upon what type of headaches you have and what the underlying cause is.

These treatments may include:

- *Soft Tissue Therapy*
- *Spinal manipulation or adjustment*
- *Low Level Laser Therapy*
- *Lifestyle Advice*

By the time a patient sees a chiropractor, he or she is usually suffering from headaches on a regular basis. If you are suffering from headaches more than two or three times a week, it is an indication that the underlying problem has been going on for some time, and that means that there won't be an "instant cure." BUT THERE WILL BE A LONG-TERM ONE!

Just as it took time for your body to become misaligned and trigger the headaches, it will take time for your body to heal properly. But with proper chiropractic care you will soon realize that your headaches are less painful and less and less frequent. Soon, they will stop altogether!

When a chiropractor designs a treatment plan, he will take into consideration a number of things, including your age, your health, the type of headaches you have, what your physical exams and X-rays and revealed, and what he or she feels will work best in combination to bring you both immediate and long-term relief.

So just what are the different types of chiropractic treatment and how do they affect headaches? Here is a breakdown of 5 of the most successful chiropractic treatments for headaches.

SOFT TISSUE THERAPY

Soft tissue therapy is the use of the hands to find and manipulate tension in the muscles and tendons of the neck and spinal region, including the shoulders if warranted. Tightening of these muscles can cause referred pain and over stimulate the nerve endings in the area. Soft tissue therapy loosens the tightness in these muscles and increases blood flow to the area to promote healing. Soft tissue massage therapy also warms and relaxes and the muscles and tendons, creating a more relaxed environment and releasing the tension so that the referred pain diminishes.

Soft tissue therapy can also be used to help break down scar tissue that has formed in the cervical area. Scar tissue that builds up in these areas can pinch nerves, decrease blood flow, and interfere with the alignment of the cervical vertebrae -- all which cause inflammation that leads to pain. With the neck so close to the head, is it any wonder that a "pain in the neck" becomes a full blown headache so often?

SPINAL MANIPULATION / ADJUSTMENT

Chiropractic manipulation focuses on correcting vertebral subluxation – the distortions in the alignment of the cervical vertebrae that lead to inflamed tissue, tightened muscles, damaged nerves, and a host of other problems that can lead to headache pain.

By carefully adjusting the vertebrae and realigning the area, the chiropractor removes the pressure and stress from the surrounding muscles and ligaments so that they can relax. This will also relieve pressure on the nerves and improve blood flow in the area if it has been constricted.

Subluxation interferes with everything from the proper flow of blood to the extremities to proper posture. If your vertebrae are consistently pulled out of alignment, the muscles and ligaments around them adjust to this, shortening on one side and lengthening on the other side in order to accommodate the

[116]

abnormality. This, in turn, causes poor posture which leads to a host of other problems.

According to a January 1999 report in the American Journal of Pain Management, "Posture and normal physiology and function are interrelated. Abnormal posture is evident in patients with chronic pain-related conditions including backache, headache, and stress-related illnesses."

Immediate relief may be felt followed by some headaches returning over the first few weeks. This is because you may have been masking the headaches with pain relievers for weeks, months, or even years. If this is the case, it can take a several weeks to "retrain" the vertebrae and surrounding tissue to their proper alignment in order to find long-term relief.

In fact, if there has been significant subluxation for a long period of time, there may be disc damage and arthritic changes due to the abnormal stress in the area. The pain caused by this can also trigger chronic headaches.

Correcting cervical subluxations provides headache relief in several ways:

- *Removing pressure from nerves*
- *Reducing muscle spasms caused by misalignment*
- *Increasing blood flow in the cervical area*
- *Preventing further damage to discs and cartilage*

Spinal adjustment is central to treating most kinds of headaches, often in combination with other types of chiropractic treatment. In most cases, the

[117]

adjustments are done manually and are painless. In some cases, you will hear a "popping" sound, which is simply the release of pressure when the bones are eased back into their proper place. You may have heard this same sound when you've cracked your knuckles. This will also relieve compression on any pinched nerve roots, which can lead to an almost immediate reduction of headache pain.

The importance of proper spinal alignment can't be underestimated, and once you get to the point where you are no longer experiencing headaches, you should consider periodic adjustments in order to maintain a healthy, properly aligned cervical region. With our busy lives, the combination of stress, physical activity, exhaustion, and simple gravity can work to create subluxations. So a periodic visit to the chiropractor is the best way to prevent today's headache and headaches in the future.

Low Level Laser Therapy

Low Level Laser Therapy (LLLT) is an astonishing new treatment method based on knowledge hundreds of years in the making. The healing properties of light have been known but not fully understood for centuries. In fact, the psychiatric community recognizes that the long-term absence of light can cause everything from depression to suppression of the body's immune system.

Low-level laser light is very specific. It is compressed light from the cold, red area of the light spectrum and is very focused and precise in nature. It travels in a straight line and is monochromatic, which means that it is a single wavelength.

The Healing Within

The unique characteristics of low level laser light enable it to penetrate the skin's surface without creating painful heat or damaging the area.

Low-level lasers work by supplying energy in the form of photons that are transmitted through the skin's surface. When these penetrate, they begin a chain reaction of responses that include:

- *An analgesic effect to reduce pain*
- *Improved blood circulation*
- *Reduction of swelling*
- *Stimulation of wound healing*
- *Stimulation of the immune system*
- *Improved cell proliferation*
- *Improved nerve function*
- *Generation of new, healthy tissue and cells*

Low Level Laser Light is applied with an instrument resembling the wand used for ultrasound. The light, although visible, isn't hot or warm, and will be applied to the area for about twenty seconds at a time. This is usually sufficient to stimulate cell response and increase blood flow to the area to encourage healing and boost the release of endorphins that aid in pain relief.

Often, the laser light will be applied to several spots along the sub-occipital region and the skull in order to reduce any inflammation, which will alleviate the headache and relax the muscles in and around the area. The cervical spine may also be treated in order to address any tension in that area.

LIFESTYLE ADVICE FOR DEALING WITH HEADACHES

As a Chiropractor, I understand that there is a delicate balance between the musculature, skeletal system, and nervous system that must be maintained for optimum health. Disturb one and you will inevitably disturb the others. That is why headaches are so common in today's society -- because we disturb our bodies' natural balance in so many ways!

There are three primary objectives to chiropractic care as it relates to a patient's complaint of headaches:

- *Stopping Acute Pain - Getting rid of the immediate headache pain and making you more comfortable*
- *Stopping Chronic Pain – Alleviating the recurring headaches and interrupting the cycle of rebound headaches that you may be caught up in*
- *Preventing Future Pain – This is the ultimate goal – giving you the tools you need to improve your overall health and understand how to care for your body so that the same problems won't return in the future.*

Proper exercise, periodic spinal adjustment, relaxation techniques, and getting enough rest are all central to maintaining your body in peak condition. Let's face it – most of us don't do enough to take care of ourselves.

In fact, most of us are seriously lacking in at least one, if not several, very important areas:

- *Getting enough sleep and rest*
- *Getting plenty of fluids during the day*

[120]

- *Using correct posture*
- *Keeping the muscles and tendons loosened and stretched properly*
- *Recognizing stress and stopping it before it affects the body*
- *Properly treating misalignment of the spine and aggravation of the nerves and blood vessels*

Headaches aren't simply temporary pains that you treat and forget about. They are red flags alerting you to underlying problems to which you need to pay close attention. Your chiropractor can help you determine what these red flags are by helping you find the proper treatments to get your body back to where it is meant to be. All of this is done so you can function at full potential once again.

You can decide for yourself how to treat your headaches. There is the traditional way or the chiropractic way. Here is a summary of each to help you decide.

The Traditional Way to Treat Headaches

- *Rebound pain*
- *Side effects like stomach irritation*
- *Chemical dependency*
- *Increasing dosages*
- *Tinnitis (ringing in the ears)*

The Chiropractic Way to Treat Headaches

- *No medications*
- *Finding and treating the cause of the headache at the source*

[121]

- *Improving overall health*
- *Preventing future headaches*

"HE/SHE TAKES MEDICINE AND NEGLECTS TO
DIET WASTES THE SKILL OF THEIR DOCTORS"
~CHINESE PROVERB

NUTRITION: THE FOUNDATION TO HEALTH

~11~

You may be asking yourself, what does nutrition have to do with chiropractic care? Well, in a nutshell: Everything! Bones, muscles, organs, and nerves – virtually every cell in the body is nourished by the foods we eat. The choices we make each time we eat are a decision to feed those cells or starve them with foods of little or no nutritive value.

The latest dietary guidelines from the U.S. Department of Agriculture have replaced the food pyramid with a more logical system that incorporates good foods in the proper quantities from each food group. It also recognizes that there isn't a one-size-fits-all approach to nutrition. Growing children and nursing mothers have far different nutritional needs for their bones and muscles than does a middle-aged man. Caloric count and make up is also different for different individuals.

The USDA has actually come up with a dietary report that gets very specific about the nutritional needs of individuals and what they recommend. Summarizing those findings, we see that more emphasis is put on lean meats, making a good portion of the grain food group choices come from whole grains, and in balancing the intake of calories against the output, or in other words, adjusting your calorie intake down if you are less active, adding calories if you are more active.

The prevalence of overweight and obesity has drastically increased in all age groups over the last few decades. An increase risk with certain health issues associated with overweight and obesity. Type II diabetes, heart disease, and certain types of cancers are associated with obesity. Obesity can increase the risk of premature death. The USDA has made the following recommendations to help prevent obesity:

- Prevent and/or reduce overweight and obesity through improved eating and physical activity behavior.
- Control total caloric intake to manage body weight. For people overweight or obese, this will mean consuming fewer calories from food and beverages.
- Increase physical activities and reduce sedentary behaviors.

Maintain appropriate caloric balance during each stage of life—childhood, adolescence, adulthood, pregnancy and breastfeeding, and older age.

Proper nutrition to sustain daily functions of the body should come from a balance diet specific to the individual. Active individuals generally need an increase in calories compare to non-active individuals due to increase of physical demands. Basically the more you exercise, the more energy you body will use to carry out normal functions of the body along the re-cooperative process due to the stress of exercise on the muscle. Here is an example of the personalize food guidelines for a 40 year old male who, in addition to his normal routine, exercises less than 30 minutes each day.

Personal Pyramid Plan

(Based on a 2400 calorie pattern)

Food Group	Serving
Grains	8 ounces
Vegetables	3 cups
Fruits	2 cups
Milk	3 cups
Meat & Beans	6.5 ounces

The specific instructions for this individual would be to aim for at least 4 whole grains each day. There should also be a variety of vegetables eaten each week. For example, it is recommended that this individual eats 3 cups of dark green vegetables each week, 2 cups of orange vegetables weekly, 3 cups of dry beans and peas a week, 6 cups of the starchy vegetables such as potatoes or corn, and 7 cups each week of other vegetables. This could include other types of lettuce, wax beans, eggplant, yellow squash, etc.

The guideline illustrates further that this individual should aim for 7 teaspoons of healthy oils a day. This might be from extra light olive oil, canola oil, etc. It is easy to get enough good oil on a salad or to stir-fry meats and vegetables.

The advice for this individual is the same for all. It is to limit the extra fats and sugars to 360 calories per day.

When you take a look at this guide, it is really not too difficult to adopt a healthy eating plan. The calories and servings are generous. The key is to eat the right types of food. If you do that, you will not be wanting for more food than is good for you to maintain a healthy weight. You will also reduce the cravings for foods that are not good for you. Keeping those portions of fats and oils under control, but not limiting them, will give a feeling of fullness and sense of satisfaction.

The new dietary guidelines also stress limiting fats, sugars, and especially sodium (salt). When you do consume the recommended small amounts of fat, the best sources are fish, nuts, and vegetable oils. You should avoid solid fats and trans fats that are hidden in the most unlikely places such as your children's snack crackers. The solid fats such as butter, margarine, and shortening, should be limited to very small quantities including those used in making other foods. It is important to read the labels on processed foods to see how much fat, sodium and sugar has been added. A can of green beans can be loaded with sodium as a preservative.

Fresh and frozen foods are always your top two choices in that order: the fresher the better. That is because once foods start to over ripen, the enzymes that are important to good health are diminished.

Eating the most whole form of the food is best too. An apple is better than apple juice because you are getting the fiber and nutrients from the peels that are not present in the juice. Plus juices often have added sugar that is not necessary and just adds extra calories and no more nutrition. Even unsweetened juices are concentrated with natural fruit sugar that is than is necessary or good.

Whole grains carry the most nutrition as well. Once a grain is broken down, it quickly loses the nutritional value. Often, the bread bakers will enrich the flour that has been stripped and bleached with nutrients, but these are never as good as the natural, whole grain.

I'm afraid much of this makes the latest fad diets seem too extreme, and in some cases, just plain unhealthy. With everything in life – whether it is food, activities, or relationships, there has to be balance. The human body is made up of many balanced systems and anything that throws it off balance will eventually lead to something less than complete wellness.

Just a word in defense of some of these low carbohydrate diets that are all the rage: there is a purpose to the plan or, if you will, a method to the madness. The intent of the Atkins diet, for example, is to achieve rapid weight loss for the morbidly obese. It is more dangerous for those people to be obese than to eat high fat, low-carb foods for a relatively short period of time. It is not meant to be a lifestyle change. The strain on the heart, muscles, bones, and joints caused by extreme obesity is life threatening and may need to be dealt with in an extreme way for the short- term. It should never be used as an ongoing way of eating for life.

Ideally, healthy eating is a life-long habit that nourishes both the mind and body with foods rich in nutrients and perfectly balanced to fight dis-ease or any kind of malaise. The following is not a diet that tells you what to eat every day, but it is a listing of the types of food choices that will provide the most nutrients to support a healthy musculoskeletal system, which in turn will keep the entire body healthy.

[128]

Some specific minerals and nutrients that are important to a strong body, especially the bones and muscles, are *calcium, magnesium, and potassium.* Also, green foods such as *alfalfa, barley, and horsetail herb* contain nutrients important to the nervous system, joints, bones, and muscles. These are not only good for a healthy back, but also help to ward off problems with high blood pressure, cholesterol, or diabetes. They create a balance in the body where each system, organ, and even cell can function at its optimal level. Then, they work together in balance one with another to maintain wellness.

Calcium

Most people are well aware that calcium is important to strengthening bones and helping prevent fractures or breaks and diseases such as osteoporosis. Something you may not realize about calcium is that when you are young your body stores calcium to be used as an adult. That is one reason why it is so important for young people, especially children, teens and those in their 20s, to get enough calcium. This calcium supply is there for the rest of their lives. It can be replaced as adults, but it isn't nearly as effective if the foundation is not established in childhood.

A strong skeletal system is what gives us good posture. Good posture is important to the prevention of subluxations that can interfere with the nerve signals transmitted from the spine that keeps every other organ and cell properly functioning. Therefore, it is easy to see why calcium is an extremely important mineral in the diet.

[129]

All of your best efforts to supply your body with enough calcium could be in vain if you unknowingly sabotage your body's ability to absorb and use the calcium. For example, if you are drinking caffeine-laden coffee with your morning calcium supplement, you are completely negating the supplement's effect. Likewise, the phosphorous in carbonated beverages hinders calcium absorption.

There are vitamins that work together with calcium to aid the absorption. These include vitamin D and vitamin K. This is why you will often find these vitamins added to milk.

Most often, we associate dairy foods with calcium. Milk, cheese, and yogurt are the highest sources of calcium in food form, but are by no means the only source. Those with allergies or intolerances to dairy products can still get plenty of calcium through whole food sources. A cup of broccoli contains 90 mg of calcium or 8% of the recommended daily value.

You can get 161 mg of calcium or 15% of the recommended daily value from just 1 ounce of cooked dried white beans. A half cup of spinach contains 122 mg of calcium which accounts for 10% of the recommended daily value, and also supplies a good amount of magnesium, which is known to be important in maintaining strong and healthy muscles.

GOOD SOURCES OF CALCIUM

Natural Food Sources	Calcium
Almonds, 2 oz	150 mg
Black Beans, 1 cup	120 mg
Part Skim Mozzarella	210 mg

[130]

Cheese, 1 oz	
Mustard Greens, ½ cup	100 mg
Soy Beans, Cooked, 1 cup	180 mg

Contrary to popular belief, infants and toddlers need less calcium than teens. Those who are 6-12 months old need only 270 mg per day. One to three year olds need 500 mg. It is the children who are growing extremely fast, between ages 9 and 18, that need 1,300 mg of calcium each day, according to the National Institutes of Health.

MAGNESIUM

Magnesium deficiency has been linked to many different back problems because of the havoc such deficiencies wreak on the muscular system. Deficiencies are also found in most patients with osteoporosis. It is clearly an important mineral and one that could be lacking from your diet.

To ensure you are getting enough magnesium, you can supplement your diet with a multi-vitamin and mineral supplement. The best way, however, to get any nutrient is from whole, fresh foods. Some of the best sources of magnesium are whole wheat bread, spinach, nuts, and black beans. These are common to the American diet and it is not difficult to have at least one serving of one of these foods each day. You will need approximately 500 mg of magnesium each day to ensure your body is not being depleted. If you cannot get it through food such as a piece of halibut with 170 mg of magnesium and a cup of spinach with 157 mg, then a supplement is important.

[131]

GOOD SOURCES OF MAGNESIUM

Food	Magnesium
Brown Rice, cooked, 1 cup	84 mg
Spinach, cooked, ½ cup	78 mg
Swiss Chard, cooked, ½ cup	75 mg
Lima Beans, cooked, ½ cup	63 mg
Avocado, 1 large	50 mg
Hazelnuts, raw, 1 oz	49 mg
Okra, cooked, ½ cup	46 mg
Black-eyed peas, cooked, ½ cup	43 mg

POTASSIUM

Potassium is an important mineral in maintaining a balance in the electrical systems of our bodies. Potassium is an electrolyte, which means it allows the ions to flow and conduct electricity inside the cells. Some enzymes also require potassium to properly perform their functions as well.

The recommended dosage of potassium each day is 2,300 mg per day for adult women and 3,100 mg per day for men. Children need slightly less. Deficiencies can lead to low bone mineral density and even stroke.

The U.S. Department of Agriculture lists some of the best food sources for potassium as *bananas, potatoes, raisins, spinach, and dried prunes.* It is easy to get enough potassium through food, given a little thought. Potassium supplements only supply 99 mg per serving. Anything higher requires a prescription and close monitoring. It can be extremely dangerous to supplement your diet with too much potassium. It is usually only necessary if you have been diagnosed with an extreme deficiency.

GOOD SOURCES OF POTASSIUM

Food	Potassium
Cod, 4 oz	580 mg
Homemade Baked Beans, 1 cup	900 mg
Potato with Skin, baked, 1 med.	925 mg
Spinach, cooked, 1 cup	840 mg
Apricots, dried, ½ cup	850 mg
Cantaloupe, ½, 5" diameter	725 mg

Bran Cereal, ½ cup	450 mg
Black-eyed peas, cooked, ½ cup	43 mg

ZINC & COPPER

Zinc is a mineral that is needed for protein synthesis. It helps in strengthening the immune system and in the formation of collagen. Taken along with copper, zinc and vitamin C work to supply the nerves with healthy nutrients.

If supplementing your diet with zinc, it is recommended that you take 50 mg per day and never more than 100 mg in a 24-hour period.

AMINO ACIDS & PROTEINS

Amino acids play an important role in maintaining strength in the cartilage and even healing torn cartilage. Amino acids are the foundation for building protein in the body. When you digest protein, the end product is amino acids. It is essential that animals, including the human animal, have proteins in their diets to live. The proteins formed from the amino acids are specifically designed to perform their necessary functions in the body. This does not have to come in the form of animal proteins by eating meat, but from a variety of low-fat and healthy sources.

Asparagine is an amino acid that is important for the central nervous system. It maintains balance within the nervous system by keeping it from

[134]

becoming too nervous or too calm. The process of converting aspargine to aspartic acid gives the brain and nerves the energy they need for metabolism.

Bones and soft tissues are also repaired with such amino acids as L-Proline. Glutamic acid works like other amino acids, as a neurotransmitter, especially to the brain and spinal cord.

VITAMINS

There are several vitamins that support a healthy back and also the connective tissue between the vertebrae and other bones in the body. A daily multivitamin can often ensure you are getting the recommended amount.

Vitamins A and E are good for providing the right amount and a balanced amount of nutrients needed to form strong and healthy bones, as well as the connective tissue. These vitamins can also help heal tissue and bone following an injury. In addition, they may be beneficial in preventing the natural deterioration of the inter-vertebral discs that can happen for individuals over the age of 40.

Vitamin B12 is important in aiding the body's ability to absorb calcium. Calcium is so important to maintaining strong bones. However, we often sabotage our calcium absorption by drinking carbonated drinks or those containing caffeine. The added benefit of vitamin B12 is that it can also aid in digestion in general.

Other B-complex vitamins do not have a direct effect on the bones but are known to strengthen the muscles, especially in the back. They are helpful in relieving stress. High stress formulas with extra B6 vitamins can be taken 3 times daily.

GLUCOSAMINE

Glucosamine is found naturally in the body in the joints. It is a classification of food that is known as an amino sugar and is formed from glucose and glutamine. It is a carbohydrate that is not used to create energy but is part of the structure of the body tissue.

People with joint trouble are often lacking in glucosamine and need to replace it in supplemental form. The added glucosamine can actually rebuild cartilage in the joints. This conclusion is the result or more than 300 clinical studies.

When taken with chondroitin sulfate, it can greatly improve osteoarthritis. This combination also helps those with tendinitis and osteoporosis.

HERBS AND PHYTO-SUPPLEMENTS

A good source of many important nutrients can be found in what are known as phyto-nutrients. Phyto refers to the plant. Green plant foods, such as barley, contain important nutrients and antioxidants. Antioxidants are those important elements that cleanse the body of cell damaging free radicals.

Some of the best ingredients for supporting a strong structural and nervous system are alfalfa herb, horsetail herb, marshmallow root, plantain herb, oat straw stem, wheat grass, and hops flowers. Alfalfa aids in assimilating minerals needed in the bones and muscles that come from the other foods you eat. So many of these foods may be processed or grown in nutrient-depleted soils so that capturing even trace amounts is important.

HORSETAIL

Horsetail herb has many minerals such as silicon, calcium, magnesium, chromium, iron, manganese and potassium. These all work together to maintain healthy joints and soft tissues in the body. They even have an astringent effect that can reduce inflammation in the joints.

MARSHMALLOW

Marshmallow root also works to reduce and heal inflammation in the tissue and contains many of the minerals found in horsetail. It can help remove excess fluid from the body and mucus.

PLANTAIN

Plantain is an herb that not only contains many nutrients, but it helps strengthen the nervous system by fighting off toxins. It also supports the digestive, urinary, and circulatory systems.

WHEAT GRASS

Wheat grass is a natural antioxidant and provides many trace nutrients. Oat straw stem contains fiber which is well known to help with digestion but also the nervous system and does hops flowers.

GOTU KOLA

Gotu Kola helps shrink tissues and can help with disorders of the connective tissues in the body. It is the nuts, roots, and seeds that are all used. It also helps eliminate excess fluid from the body and has many healthy benefits including stimulating the central nervous system.

The list of beneficial herbs for the body is almost endless. Here is a partial listing of herbs that can benefit the bones and joints by strengthening tissues. Many can be used in your everyday meal preparation or in supplement form:

- *Alfalfa*
- *Black Cohosh*
- *Cat's Claw*
- *Cayenne*
- *Dandelion*
- *Garlic*

- *Ginger*
- *Peppermint*
- *Sarsaparilla*
- *Thyme*
- *Wild oregano*

The brain and nervous system are also nourished by specific herbs:

[138]

- *Billberry*
- *Blessed thistle*
- *Celery*
- *Chamomile*

- *Fennel*
- *Rosemary*
- *Wintergreen*

Finally, the muscles receive sustenance from:

- *Eucalyptus*
- *Ginger*
- *Kava kava*
- *Licorice*
- *Skullcap*
- *Wild yam*

Most of these phyto-nutrients are not found in high enough quantities in foods and require taking an herbal supplement. This can be in the form of a pill, powder, or tea for equally effective benefits.

WATER

Anyone who has tried to lose weight or manage some kind of health problem naturally, such as high cholesterol or high blood pressure, has undoubtedly been told by their health care provider to drink more water. Why is that? Water doesn't really contain any nutritional elements and it doesn't always taste great. So why is water so important to good health?

The primary reason that water is necessary to good health is found in the fact that our bodies are made up mostly of water, about 70%, and need plenty of it to function properly. Water also acts as a catalyst to other nutrients and especially antioxidants doing their job. Water is essential to maintaining proper blood volume and in cleansing toxins from the body.

There are serious conditions that also result from an insufficient intake of water. Dehydration is one that is most well-known, but it is only the beginning of other organs shutting down from performing their functions.

If you have ever skimped on your water intake for a day, you have probably felt lethargic and most likely even had a pounding headache. Water can relieve the headache, as well as contribute aid to many other healing processes. Here is a list by Dr. George Grant from the International Academy of Wellness:

[140]

Water helps to:

- *Relieve/Prevent: lower back pain, Chronic Fatigue Syndrome, headaches, migraines, asthma, allergies, colitis, rheumatoid arthritis, depression, hypertension, cholesterol, hangovers, neck pain, muscle pain, joint pain, bloating, constipation, ulcers, low energy levels, stomach pain, confusion, and disorientation.*

- *Maintain: muscle tone, weight loss, clear and healthy skin.*

- *Regulate: body temperature, remove toxins and wastes, cushion and lubricate joints, decrease risk of kidney stones, protect tissues, organs and the spinal cord from shock and damage.*

- *Assist In: the digestion & absorption of food, and in transporting oxygen and nutrients to the cells.*

YOUR pH BALANCE

Just as there should be balance in our activities in life and the types of foods we eat, there needs to be balance between acidity and alkalinity in our systems. The pH balance is important to so many aspects of health. Here I'd like to talk about the amazing benefits of alkalinity in our diets. To get a better grasp on the subject, it helps to first understand some of the vocabulary.

The first question to address is, "What is alkalinity?" Alkalinity, which refers to the system of pH, is determined by the concentration of hydrogen in a substance. This can be water, food, or blood. On a scale from 1-14, a pH of 7 is considered neutral, while 14 is extremely alkaline, and 0 is pure acid. The body is designed to be slightly neutral. When it is not, the effects on the body can be remarkable.

Just like body temperature, the body prefers a specific pH to create healthy reactions. The pH of the intercellular fluid affects every cell in the human body. The entire metabolic pathway is dependent on the pH environment.

When pH is out of the desirable range, it can be the source of a vast number of degenerative conditions. The problem with the pH system is that cellular processes are constantly creating acidic waste. That is why it is so important to add alkalinity to the system to support the body. Actually, it is essential to counteract the effects of metabolism in our body.

Researchers are now stating that pH balance is the most important aspect of a healthy body and a long, disease-free life. Degenerative conditions such as arthritis can be caused by pH imbalances, due to the fact that when the body is in an acidic environment, the body begins to deplete the alkaline stores in our body. Those stored alkaline resources can be the calcium and other minerals that are used as a buffer in the body. Therefore, an imbalance of alkalinity can create a condition favorable to the growth of yeast, viruses, bacteria, and other harmful organisms – even cancer.

It is important to understand that even small fluctuations in body temperature could lead to death. It is also important to realize the significance in the maintenance of the pH system. If, for example, the pH of a person would drop to 6.95, this condition could lead to serious health risks, such as death or coma.

[142]

When we speak of internal cell metabolism leading to acid production, we are really more concerned about the more dangerous scenario which plagues a vast majority of society. It is the effects that our diet has on our blood chemistry. Normal blood chemistry is 20 percent acid and 80 percent alkaline, which, in turn, creates the acid-base balance. Food choices, especially over a long period of time, can keep blood chemistry at dangerous levels of acidity for too long.

When you decrease the alkalinity in the blood even slightly, the ability of the blood to transport carbon dioxide out of the cell gets reduced. This will result in an accumulation of acid in the tissues. This condition is known as hypo-alkalinity or acidosis. This condition can seriously interfere with the functions of the organs and systems of the body.

The effects of acid in the body, therefore, can be devastating. Research now shows that this type of environment within the blood can affect the following areas or create certain conditions including:

- *Digestion*
- *Obesity*
- *Cardiovascular function*
- *Kidney disease*
- *Mental and neurological issues*
- *Arthritic conditions*

Digestive Issues

The pancreas regulates the pH balance by producing HCL and buffers. When the pH of any of these areas is compromised, food can't be properly broken down and absorbed.

[143]

It is estimated that 100 million Americans suffer from digestive problems, and 10 million are hospitalized for it. Much of this may be attributed to an imbalance of pH caused by diet.

Some believe that in order to treat cases of acid reflux one can consume raw potatoes. The reason raw potatoes are thought to help is their alkaline nature. The potatoes also are good because of their enzymatic properties which are essential for the breakdown of food in the digestive system.

According to the National Institute of Health, obesity is on the rise, and there is a direct correlation between the overall quality of our foods and the nation's epidemic. Listen to these scary statistics. Nationally, obesity rates have increased sharply from 12% to 19% during the 1990's. In the state of Washington, however the increase was even more significant during the same period. How is this happening?

Dr. Robert Young in his book, *The pH Miracle*, describes fat as the body's defense mechanism, designed to carry away acids from vital organs to try to protect them. Weight issues, as explained in his book, can also be due to exhaustion of the adrenal and the thyroid glands. Again, when the body is acidic, it tries to neutralize the potency of the acid by diluting it leading to water retention.

Cardiovascular Disease and Acid

Cardiovascular disease is the number one killer in this country, claiming more than 850,000 people a year. A whopping 37% of those people, who died of this condition, didn't have any symptoms prior to their death! How can this be?

[144]

Again, we live in a society that lives off of symptoms as an indicator of health, yet this condition, which kills more people in this country, is silent in almost 40% of the cases. This is truly an epidemic!

Just what causes fatty plaque to form along the walls of the arteries? How is it that patients with angioplasty have clean arteries, then six months later, have a relapse, in which there arteries are filled up again?

Researchers may have come up with the culprit: Cytomegalovirus which located in the walls of the blood vessels. There are several studies that support the theory of the virus being present and the unexplained onset of plaque. In one study, 75 percent of those patients who were infected with the virus had a recurrence of plaque. Only 8 percent of those with no virus had a recurrence, an astonishing finding, considering this is not talked about at all in the media.

That's right; no one is telling us this. What is so amazing about this finding is that this virus, as well as other viruses and bacteria, only thrives in acidic environments. In reference to this fact, it is important to remember the famous German pathologist Rudolf Virchow (1821-1902), who came to the realization after researching the germ theory his entire life, said, "If I could live my life over again, I would devote it proving that germs seek their natural habitat – diseased tissue. For example, mosquitoes seek the stagnant water but do not cause the pool to become stagnant."

Another condition that plagues people with heart condition is inflammation of the arterial walls. According to the April 1999 issue of the New England Journal of Medicine, men whose arteries were inflamed for several years were three times more likely to have heart attacks and two times more likely to have strokes as individuals whose arteries were not inflamed. Now, what is so interesting about this finding is that an acidic environment causes scratches and tears on the interior of the blood vessel wall. The effect of this is an immune response to defend the walls which, unfortunately, creates an inflammatory response due to the immuno-response, causing blood to enter into the walls as a defense mechanism. In essence, this reaction is very similar to what happens when there is bodily injury from accidents. It creates an inflammatory response. Amazing isn't it?

High Cholesterol

Is cholesterol the bad guy it has been labeled as? Perhaps not. The late Dr. G.E. Barnes conducted a study using 50,000 autopsies of people who died in World War II when saturated fats like meat and butter were very scarce. The findings were very surprising. They indicated that there was a high percentage of hardening of the arteries despite a low cholesterol diet. This should shed some light on the fact that dietary cholesterol may not be the only culprit in excessive cholesterol levels – the kind that lead to heart disease.

Could high cholesterol actually be due to the acidic environment that causes the viruses and bacteria to proliferate, causing an immune response which in turn causes inflammation and subsequently hardening of the arteries? It is something to think about and investigate before starting a life-long dependency on statin drugs with their sometimes serious side effects.

Kidney Disease

Acid also plays a significant role in kidney disorders. Within the kidneys lie millions and millions of cells known as nephrons. These tiny cells are designed

[146]

to filter waste and allow for the absorption of essential fluids and nutrients back into the system. Specifically, the nephrons remove waste that may consist of water, urea, uric acid, and ammonia.

Now, if the nephrons were to process a small amount of uric acid, there would be virtually no kidney failure known to mankind. Yet, with the American diet, we may be poisoning our inner terrain with excessive levels of acid, making it difficult to filter and process the uric acid, which is a byproduct of nitrogen-based foods. You should therefore, avoid foods that are high in purines. These foods include:

- *Beer or other alcoholic beverages*
- *Yeast*
- *Legumes (peas and dried beans)*
- *Organ meats (kidneys, liver)*
- *Meat extracts (such as ingredients in gravies)*
- *Spinach, asparagus, cauliflower*

Am I saying that you can't consume any products that are high or moderately high in purines? Absolutely not: what I am saying is that in order for you to consume these foods, you must be aware of the consequence of consuming them without countering the effects with alkaline-based foods. Many of the above foods have other nutritional benefits. That may be why, perhaps, a tradition of "meat and potatoes" is a part of so many cultures. The potatoes are alkaline and can count the impact of acidic foods such as meat gravy or the yeast from bread.

The unfortunate part of dealing with kidney disorders is that the kidneys do not show as much versatility as we would like them to have. As with the case of the cardiovascular system, when the nephrons have to filter away the excessive acid, they are compromised by the scraping and scratching effects that the acids have on the micro blood vessel walls.

With the blood vessels it takes years, if not decades, to see the effect of plaque buildup in normal blood vessel walls. This is not the case with the nephrons. When nephrons are compromised, and the hormonal system of the body kicks in, it begins to increase fluid flow through the nephrons which will ease the strain on the cells.

With that however, comes an increase in blood pressure. The medical community responds to this by counteracting the effects of the rise in blood pressure with a diuretic. This further adds excessive strain to the kidneys to filter the solid materials out of the blood. The kidney is a very sensitive organ. It does not have the regenerative abilities of the liver.

Incidentally, new research from Georgetown University shows that rats treated with a steady diet of dark green vegetables have stimulated the production of new alveoli (new air sacs). However, research does not show these properties to be found in the kidney.

Neurological Impact

Acid further impacts the mind and neurological system. Again, whenever you begin to alter the pH terrain, you can alter processing and functions within the body. When the brain has within its environment excessive acidic waste, it can be responsible for the swelling of the corpus collusum and of the ventricles. This data was reported by Fred Bookstein of the University of Michigan's medical center in the examination of schizophrenics.

To make matters worse, symptoms of fear, anxiety, and other intense disempowering emotions cause the production of a hormone known as cortisol. When the release of cortisol is prolonged, it can have a detrimental impact on the brain cells in the hippocampus (a part of the limbic system where memories are stored). The problem with this scenario is that it can lead to further issues. Whenever the neurons are being compromised with excessive acidic waste, it causes them to die off, creating further acidic production which is thus carried off by the capillaries into general circulation. This excessive acidic waste comes across as solidified alkaline minerals which are deposited into organ systems, thus giving rise to degenerative conditions.

Why is this not being told to us? The reason is that neuroscientists do not want to believe that chemistry improvement via nutritional remedy is the answer. It can't be; it would denounce all their work and research. After all, according the World Health Organization, depression is as common as the common cold. It's the third most common illness in the world after infectious disease and heart disease.

Depression is considered the 4th to the 10th most frequent diagnosis made by the family doctor. It is disturbing to know that in this country by December 1995 there had already been reported 35,230 cases of adverse reactions to the mother of all antidepressants – Prozac. These side effects included hallucination, aggression, hostility, assault, manslaughter, and suicide, resulting in a total of 2,394 deaths! Something is wrong with this picture.

I'm not saying that there are not cases in which there are definite chemical imbalances, but I believe the vast majority of prescriptions are given as a magical pill that will solve their problems. Whenever I have a patient in my office that is on an anti-depressant, I invariably ask them how happy they are with their life. I ask them how happy they are with the direction of their life. I ask them what they picture for their future. Is it a positive anticipation that they have toward it? The vast majority of them tell me that they are not happy with their life. You see most people that are not feeling well emotionally, in my opinion, are giving themselves a sign that something must change.

Dissatisfaction can be a powerful ally when you are aware of its purpose and how it is trying to serve you. Again, as stated, I do believe that there are people with emotional issues due to chemical imbalance including issues with serotonin and other chemicals. It is my opinion that a complete analysis of their diet, for the detection of an over-acidic diet and other nutritional issues, is necessary.

Arthritis and pH

There is also a connection between arthritic changes and acid in our body. Here's an interesting fact: the body needs calcium for its alkaline properties for healthy nerve and blood function more so than for the skeletal system. We always assume calcium's most important job is build bones.

Excessive acid in the diet will extract calcium from the bones. Again we need to remind ourselves that calcium is an alkalizing forming agent, able to neutralize the effects of an acidic environment. The problem with this scenario is

[150]

that when calcium combines with the acid, it creates a solid – calcium carbonate, and this alkalizing compound unfortunately is deposited in the bone joints and vertebrae.

Osteoporosis works along the same premise. However, one thing to realize is that if you are prone to osteoporosis being a female, or because you don't exercising, or a combination of both, it would be very, very wise for you to not consume soda. Yes, you read right – SODA! Why is that? In a nutshell, soft drinks are extremely acidic. They have a pH of 2.5, which can be disastrous to the body. So stay clear from soda and don't even consider trying to justify it. It is terrible for you!

If you are prone to brittle bones, you must increase your intake of alkaline foods that can replenish your calcium levels. Now please be aware that in order for your body to properly absorb calcium, it must have cofactors such as magnesium and vitamin D.

One side note about osteoporosis: If you are not moving -- if you are not exercising -- you will also increase your odds of having this condition due to the law of demand. Meaning if you do not put healthy stress on the body, the body will find more important areas in it where it can use the calcium since it's not being used for the support of bone mass. In order to keep calcium in the bones, the bones must be challenged.

So how do you determine if you are acidic anyway? There are various ways by which you can determine your pH. The first way is by taking the pH of your urine. Specifically, the first urine of the morning tells you how your body handled the food you consumed the day before. Testing your pH is very simple.

[151]

The first thing you need to do is get the proper pH strip supply. I recommend either pH ion or go to the pH miracle.us for supplies. What you want to be looking for are strips that show pH levels in increments of 0.2, otherwise you will need to see a large change in your pH to see anything different on the pH strip. pH strips work by measuring acid on a numerical scale. Each whole number increase or decrease corresponds to a tenfold change in your pH.

Therefore, the first order of business the day you check your pH is to wake up in the morning and catch some urine in a small clean container. Then test the pH of the urine by placing the strip into the urine. The change in color will be immediate. Then compare the color of the strip to the color coordinated pH range paper provided with the strips to see what the results are.

This first test will check your baseline pH. The next step is to determine your alkaline reserves. This is done by challenging your body with an environment of acid. This will determine to what extent you have alkalinity reservation. To do this, you will need to expose your body to a 2-day acidic diet, rich in proteins, hamburgers, breads, and very few vegetables.

I hope at this point that you are not saying that you don't really need to change anything with your diet, because this represents what you normally eat! This type of diet is highly acidic and needs to be used just to see what type of alkaline reserve you have.

Here is a summary of what you are to do for the next three days:

Day 1

[152]

Take the baseline standard of your pH by checking your urine in the morning. Only consume acid producing foods so as to challenge your alkaline reserves; foods such as breads, meats, chicken, etc. Throughout this process, please remember to drink plenty of water.

Day 2

Repeat of what you did on day one.

Day 3

You can resume your normal intake of foods. Just remember to take your urine pH level first thing in the morning.

Analyzing the Results

If after the two days, it shows that the pH of your urine is high, you may have a problem. If the pH is low, you have alkaline reserves.

If your pH was between 6.8 and 8.0, it means that your diet for the last 2 days challenged the body and determined that it had very little alkaline reserves, if any. How do we know this? It's simple. When your body is in an acidic environment, specifically the acid of urine, it must be neutralized. The body uses minerals to do the job. If, however, the body does not have sufficient levels, it will depend on ammonia which is a very powerful alkaline compound. Therefore, it will give you the illusion through the reading of your urine that indeed you are alkaline. That is not the case.

So, now what should you do? The key is to transition in a way that a body can gently adapt to the changes. The body has grown accustomed to your present dietary habits. The last thing it needs is to be shocked. Therefore, the key is to replace one acid with one alkaline. For example replace peanut butter with almond butter or replace cow's milk with soy or rice milk.

Here is a list of food groups that constitute acid and alkaline.

Highly Acidic	Highly Alkaline
Soda	Potatoes
Coffee	Spinach
Fish	Turnip greens
Meat	Dandelion greens
Beans	Orange juice
Most grains	Bananas
Sour cream	Figs
Yogurt	Tomato juice
Eggs	Mineral supplements

It may surprise you to see citrus juices or tomato juice on the alkaline side of the list. These foods start out being acidic, but the way they are processed in digestion leaves a residue that is alkaline, therefore they are classified as alkaline foods with all of the alkaline benefits.

One side note on the reason why we should consume green leafy vegetables: It is that they contain a much needed mineral known as magnesium. This mineral is considered a co-factor in over 300 enzymatic processes, without which leads to serious complications within the body.

There are over 200 published clinical studies documenting the need for proper magnesium intake. Deficiency in the body can lead to very serious

[154]

problems according to a recent article by Dr. Sidney Baker. A deficiency in this mineral can lead to muscle soreness, twitches, cramps, back ache, neck pain, as well as tension headache and even TMJ dysfunction.

This is just covering its impact on the muscular system. Magnesium plays an important role in the central nervous system. A deficiency in this area can cause insomnia, anxiety, hyperactivity and restlessness, or panic attacks. When pertaining to the peripheral nervous system, symptoms can be numbness, tingling, and other abnormal sensations.

With reference to the cardiovascular system, the research does show that deficiencies of magnesium may cause symptoms such as heart palpitations, high blood pressure, or angina due to spasms of the coronary arteries.

So as you can see this mineral is essential for vital function. Why do I bring this up? I bring it up because not only do raw green leafy vegetables provide the body with a powerful alkaline bath, they also provide magnesium and other cancer fighting agents in the plant. Again the reason why you want to consume vegetables is that they contain chlorophyll. Within the center of this molecule lies the magnesium molecule waiting to be utilized by the body.

"WATER IS THE MOST NEGLECTED NUTRIENT IN YOUR DIET BUT ONE OF THE MOST VITAL"

~KELLY BARTON

WELLNESS AND PREVENTION

~12~

It is much easier to prevent than to cure. Think about it. It really is a no-brainer. If you can keep yourself healthy through diet, exercise, and controlling stress, you are much better off than having to deal with the dis-ease or conditions created through poor choices.

Choosing to live a healthy lifestyle and care not only for your spine but for every part of the body and mind should be a relatively simple choice. No one wants to be unhealthy. No one wants pain. No one wants to be limited in their movement or abilities, either physical or mental.

Sometimes it is only a matter of knowing what to do and how to do it. You know what you want the end results to be, but you are just not sure how to get from point A to point B. This is where I come in. As a chiropractor, personally and professionally, I have made a commitment to educate myself and others on how to get the most from their body and, in turn, get the most out of living a healthy, pain-free and illness-free life.

Now, I am not saying that if you always eat right, exercise, and lift safely and move properly you will never ever get sick or injured. All that I am saying is that you increase the likelihood that your body will be prepared to handle the external forces placed upon your body. With good nutrition and exercise for example, you are naturally creating a stronger immune system against toxins in the air, viruses brought on and spread by others, and you are creating a strong defense against a myriad of diseases.

To build and protect yourself against injury, exercise and diet build strong bones and muscles. An impact-related injury then is less likely to damage them. A spine that is kept in alignment through preventative chiropractic care is then more easily corrected through a minor adjustment following an injury. Again, you are keeping the spine free from blockage or subluxation that can prevent the body from correcting that which is wrong and keeping itself healthy. Yes, an ounce of prevention is worth a pound of cure has never been more true than when it comes to your health and well-being.

MANAGING STRESS

Far too little emphasis is placed today on the reality that emotional stress, mental trauma, and phobias can cause real and damaging physical reactions and responses in the body. When you are emotionally stressed there are subtle changes in posture which strain the joints and muscles. This leaves them susceptible to injury. Mental stress can even cause compression in spinal joints.

There are many successful ways to reduce stress. One method may work perfectly for one person, while another person needs to try something different. Controlling stress is an extremely individual process. No two people go about it exactly the same way. The key here is to find out what works for you and apply it whenever necessary.

There are some basic categories to reducing stress. Within one of these you will probably find a more specific method that works for you. The goal is control the mind's stress with a mental or physical activity that brings about real physical changes such as slowing the heart rate, lowering blood pressure, releasing

[158]

muscle tension, etc. Any physical change brought about by mental stresses such as deadlines, work, or financial worries, can also be changed back to a more desirable state through stress-reduction techniques.

STRESS REDUCING EXERCISES

There are so many benefits to exercise, one of which is to reduce stress. Exercise does not have to entail a lengthy visit to the local gym or changing into specific clothing and formally doing calisthenics. Exercise is simply moving in a way that gets the heart pumping and the blood flowing so that endorphins can be released. Endorphins are those chemicals that make you feel a sense of elation and a sense of physical and mental wellness. Some people refer to it as a natural "high."

Here are some great exercises that require no equipment except some good shoes and very little preparation. They can be done on a moments notice to reduce stress and refresh both the mind and body.

- Take a brisk 20-minute walk in the sunshine
- Walk the dog at a slower pace for 30 minutes
- House and yard work. You need to do these chores anyway; why not use them to break up periods of work at the computer or desk to exercise large muscle groups and clear your mind?

Making time to reduce stress is equally as important as these spur of the moment breaks. If you set aside a time each day to mentally and physically prepare yourself for the day, or to unwind at the end of a stressful day, then you will have something to look forward to each day. I promise you that if you make this time, you will begin to look forward to it each day as your period of renewal. It will become well-deserved "me time." You will come to protect it as an important part of the day and miss it when you don't take the time to de-stress.

During this stress reduction time you will set aside for yourself, you can either exercise or engage in some other form of stress reduction. Here are some other great activities that require little skill or preparation:

- Mediation
- Tai Chi
- Yoga
- Stretching exercises
- Motivational or inspirational reading (remember it doesn't have to be physical. Nourishing the mind can reduce physical stress symptoms.

MEDITATION

Meditation is actually a factor in improving the function of the immune system. Studies conducted at the University of Wisconsin confirmed this fact.

The study used a meditation technique called mindfulness-based stress reduction. Forty-eight healthy people were divided into two groups. They received meditation training over the course of eight weeks and in addition received a vaccine for influenza.

Evaluation of blood samples at the four and eight-week marks indicated that there were increased antibodies at significant levels in the patients practicing the mediation techniques. This increase is a sure sign that the body's immune

[160]

system is strong and healthy. Of even more importance is the fact that a healthy immune system is central to enjoying overall good health.

There are meditation techniques you can use at any time and in any place. However, the most effective meditative practice to relieve mental and physical stress is achieved when you can devote a specific amount of time to removing yourself from all external disruptions.

It does not have to take up a lot of time, perhaps 15 to 20 minutes, but it should be a quiet time in a place where other people or the telephone cannot disturb you.

MINDFULNESS-BASED STRESS REDUCTION

The Mindfulness-Based Stress Reduction Technique (MBSR) for meditation was developed at the University of Massachusetts Medical Center in 1979. It is still widely practiced and regarded as effective today.

Proponents of MBSR, after more than 20 years of research, have concluded that the results include everything from an increased ability to relax to improved self-esteem. They have also witnessed long term reductions in physical and psychological symptoms.

The technique works by first increasing awareness in all aspects related to the individual. This includes a sense of your physical being and mental self. It is based on the premise that we already have within us this knowledge of self, but must bring it to the point of awareness.

[161]

MBSR is credited with helping those who have chronic pain or illness, headaches, high blood pressure, sleep and intestinal problems, and anxiety disorders. It also benefits those who have stresses related to work, home, or finances. These external stresses can lead to the physical health problems already able to be treated by practicing MBSR.

The technique works by being mindful of surrounding sounds, including your own breathing. It focuses on rhythm and patterns related to how we react to specific situations. Included in the technique are stretching exercises for the purpose of coming to a mindful and aware state of being.

ACUPUNCTURE

This ancient Chinese method of inserting very fine needles into the body to induce a physiological response is more than 4,000 years old. It relates directly to the idea of so many other alternative medicines, including chiropractic, that the body has an energy running through it. In Chinese, the energy is referred to as Qi and is pronounced "chee." Qi has a direct impact on the balance and wellness of all systems in the body.

Just like with nerve signals, Qi can have interference that prevents optimal health. The goal of the acupuncturist is to remove the obstacles, just like the chiropractor removes the subluxation. Perhaps that is why many chiropractors also incorporate acupuncture or the non-invasive, more massage-like form, acupressure, into their practices.

Acupuncture also has a map of the body where certain stimulus points are related to organs and systems in the body. Sometimes acupuncture needles are inserted with a small electrical impulse added to further stimulate the area and remove the interference.

The energy is believed to flow down the pathways called meridians. The meridians need to be free from interference or obstructions and in balance in order to achieve optimal health.

TAI CHI

Tai Chi is all about balance and harmony in the body. It goes very well with the chiropractic way of health care, as both strive for that balance.

The balanced state within Tai Chi is often referred to as Yin & Yang. The premise behind both Tai Chi and Chinese medicine is to increase the natural energy in the body. In chiropractic, we refer to that natural energy as innate intelligence. When Chi is not flowing properly in the body, there is a feeling of not being well. Conversely, a free flowing Chi within oneself leads to a feeling of being well.

Tai Chi can be considered both a physical and mental exercise. In order to awaken or release energy flow, specific movements and positions are enacted. Breathing techniques and exercises go hand in hand with the movements. These form sets and activities have different purposes, but all improve muscle tone, balance, flexibility, mobility, and work to improve concentration all through releasing greater energy flow.

Tai Chi can be done at home with videos to guide you. There are more and more classes and schools specific to the Chinese method also popping up as people become more knowledgeable of the art and it becomes more accepted as a viable method of maintaining good health.

YOGA

Yoga has many different applications for good health. There are specific movements, called poses, which can help with blood pressure, insomnia, osteoporosis, and especially stress. In fact, there are dozens of poses known to help with even more aliments and the prevention of them.

To perform yoga, the only "equipment" you need is an open mind and perhaps a good foam mat. This helps make some of the poses more comfortable. Loose clothing won't restrict your movements and is also important.

THOSE WHO THINK THEY HAVE NOT TIME FOR

BODILY EXERCISE WILL SOONER OR LATER

HAVE TO FIND TIME FOR ILLNESS."

~EDWARD STANLEY

DAILY ACTIVITIES TO IMPROVE QUALITY OF LIFE
~13~

Exercise is not only important to good cardiovascular health and muscle tone but it is also significant to posture. When muscle tone in the back is good, we naturally have better posture and without thinking about it. The muscles in the back are what help to hold the spine erect. Our shoulders are relaxed and not up around our ears when we have good muscle tone and when we free ourselves from stress through methods such as relaxation techniques and exercise. All without thinking we are naturally assuming a better posture and it is a comfortable position.

THE CORRELATION OF MUSCLE STRENGTH & BONE DENSITY

Remember your mother telling you to sit up straight or your back will stick that way? It wasn't that the spine would permanently grow into a slouched position, but the muscle tone would become so weak that it couldn't hold the spine up.

A great deal of research has gone into the skeletal and muscular effects of exercise. In a conference on osteoporosis prevention, Dr. Robert A. Marcus reported on the impact of exercise on both muscle tone and bone density, and how that impacted overall health. The research revealed that Bone Mineral Density (BMD) didn't necessarily increase with moderate exercise, but without it, it most assuredly decreased. It took the very high impact activities such as jumping and running to increase BMD. However, even just standing helps hold on to current levels of BMD.

Even without increasing BMD, muscle strength can be increased with exercise. This is especially important for the elderly who cannot engage in most other activities that promote increases in BMD. Just by toning muscles, especially leg muscles, even those in the 90s are able to reduce the risk of serious injury if they fall, even without increasing BMD.

The only group of people in the research conducted on BMD that had differing results was children. The time when a person is usually most active is childhood. Children are able to build a reserve of BMD that provides benefits throughout life. An inactive child might have problems with BMD as an adult. In order for any adult, however, to maintain good BMD, they must continuously exercise throughout their life.

Some good exercises for strengthening the back and improving posture include strengthening many other muscle groups. Some of these are:

- *Abdominal*
- *Hamstrings*
- *Quadriceps*
- *Gluteus*
- *Front Neck*
- *Scapula (shoulder blade) supporting muscles*

There are many effective exercises for each muscle group and for any level of fitness. Any exercise that flexes the muscle and stretches it gently is good. When doing an exercise, it is better to do shorter repetitive sets than to completely exhaust the muscle. Doing 10 or 12 repetitions is good for each group to start. Then you can gradually increase the number as the muscles become conditioned.

You never want to overwork the muscles. It will just lead to soreness, at the very least, and even more serious injury. If, for example, you were to lift weights using one muscle group, you would want to rest those muscles for a day before repeating those exercises. This is especially true as you get into heavier weights for resistance.

PILATES

There are different types of exercises, some as old as 5000 years that provide good strength to muscles. Pilates is a back friendly method of toning that focuses on all of the large muscle groups. It not only strengthens muscles, but increases flexibility in a gentle and effective way. It is an easy program to adopt no matter at what fitness level you are starting.

Joseph Pilates developed the exercise program as a way to first of all strengthen his own body. He was a sickly child and unable to do many of the other childhood activities others enjoyed. During World War I, he further tested his strengthening concepts as a nurse and used his exercises to increase mobility in disabled veterans.

Today there are over 500 different Pilates exercises that focus not only on strengthening the core muscles, but centering and breathing. Together, with concentration, those who implement Pilates exercises will quickly see improved posture and flexibility, along with the ability to balance in positions holding their center of gravity.

[168]

ERGONOMICS

Ergonomics is a science which studies the way in which the human body responds to the forces of nature put on the body through physical activity. In Greek the terms ergon (work) and nomoi (natural laws) are combined to create the English word, ergonomics.

The goal of ergonomics is to reduce injuries by being aware of how the everyday activities in which we engage affect our joints and muscles. There are three basic rules to ergonomics that, if applied, would greatly reduce stress or repetitive movement injuries common in the workplace. They include changing positions often to other healthy positions, using the largest muscle group for any type of force exerted, and only working joints to the mid-point of their range of motion.

When speaking of ergonomics, it is important to understand that there is static work and then there is force. The static work refers to those tasks where you are required to maintain the same position or small movement for extended periods of time. This may include typing, standing at lab bench while bending over a microscope, or sitting in a truck with one hand on the steering wheel day after day.

Force as it relates to ergonomics is all about how much the muscles have to work. If the wrong muscles are used for the job, then there can be injury. This is not limited to lifting heavy objects, but can even include flexing the neck muscles to bend the head forward or backward from the upright position. This action alone, adds four times the force on the lower neck vertebra. So if you have a job where your head is bent down looking over paperwork, you are putting excessive force on your neck.

The way to counteract the impact of static work and force on the muscles and bones is to become conscious of each movement and change positions frequently throughout the day. Also using the largest appropriate muscles for any task minimizes the risk of injury.

Ergonomics takes thought. Thinking about your posture and the different positions you assume in any given task is not something we naturally do. We simply try to be comfortable. Really the only time we give thought to our position or posture is when we are uncomfortable. We then seek to change to a more relaxed way of feeling good and relieving the discomfort. Again, there is not much thought given to the process, we just move until it feels good.

Since we naturally put little thought into ergonomics, doctors and scientists have been doing it for us. They have worked to create tools and methods to ease the stresses we put on our joints and muscles. Some of the most notable inventions of the 20th century included the foam strip at the base of computer keyboards which raises the wrists to a better position for the wrist joints. This reduced the cases of carpal tunnel syndrome experienced by typists who often spend several hours each day in that position.

Likewise, office chairs with lumbar support encouraged better posture for desk dwellers. We also saw an increase in the use of headsets for receptionists who, prior to that, would often cradle the telephone receiver between their ear and shoulder while taking notes. In many workstations you will see the semi-seated workstation. This is a type of chair where you are neither sitting nor standing. It keeps the lower back aligned with the rest of the back and actually promotes good posture. That, in turn, relieves pressure on the spine and alleviates back pain, especially in the lower back.

Ergonomics goes even further into our everyday lifestyle than for that of office workers or others who engage in repetitive movement for the majority of their day. Simple changes in the way we carry out everyday activities can make a difference in how well our backs and joints are protected. Each applies the three basic principles of ergonomics stated earlier: adopting differing positions; using the largest muscles for a task; and staying within the mid-point in a joint's range of motion.

APPLYING ERGONOMIC PRINCIPLES

Lifting

Lifting anything applies the rule of ergonomics related to using the largest muscle group. The group, erogonomics.org, refers to this as the "largest appropriate muscle group." Obviously you wouldn't use your forearm to push a light switch when an "appropriate" muscle is the finger. To lift heavier objects or move heavier items is where this principle is mostly concerned.

Most people are well aware that if you lift a heavy box by bending over and pulling up with the arms, your back is going to take the brunt of the weight, and by doing most of the work, risk the greatest injury to the back. That is why movers will wear thick belts. This supports the back and actually prevents the back from doing the work. The largest muscles in the body are found in the upper legs. These should always take most of the weight and exertion when lifting. Here are some important tips when lifting:

- *Bend down, not over.* If you are squatting, then you must naturally use your legs to rise and lift the object with them.

- *Work with a partner.* Whenever possible, lighten the load by getting someone else to lift with you.

- *Keep the back vertical.* When the trunk is horizontal it actually adds hundreds of pounds of pressure on just a small section of the spine that then acts as a fulcrum.

- *Keep objects you are lifting close to the body.* The stress on the spine is exponentially related to the distance the object being lifted.

- *When lifting a heavy object from above your head to lower it,* get up close on a step stool to avoid holding the weight overhead with your arms. Again, closer is better when lifting.

Carrying Children

Many of the same principles that apply to lifting heavy objects apply to lifting and carrying children. You will often times see an infant or toddler perched on a mother's hip. Think about her posture. Is her trunk vertical or is it skewed to one side to compensate for the added weight on her hip?

There are many great devices to help make carrying children easier and safer. The best and safest choices are ones that allow the weight to be evenly distributed and that keep the trunk and spine in a good vertical alignment. An example of this is the over-the-shoulder sling that holds an infant up to almost chest level in front of the parent. This shouldn't be used for extended periods of time, or after the baby gets to be so heavy that the parent is forced to bend forward or backward to compensate for the added weight.

When carrying older or heavier children for any length of time, it is best to carry them on your back, piggyback style. A back pack carrier is good for walks or hikes because its waist straps distribute more weight to the hips than the back – again, using the larger muscles to carry the load.

When lifting a child out of a crib or pack 'n play, get as close to the side as possible. If the sides to the crib can be lowered, always do that first so that you do not have to lift above your head as much. Wrap your arms around the child's midsection with one arm supporting their lower body, and bring them close to you before lifting upward. You may have to bend over to cradle an infant lying on his back, but you can still bring him close to you before moving upward.

Standing up

When was the last time you thought about how you were getting out of bed in the morning or standing up from sitting in a chair? You probably never give it any thought unless it is uncomfortable or even painful. There are methods of standing up that relieve pain and prevent strain or injury to the back. Some of these apply the ergonomic principle of staying within the mid-range of joint motion.

Start the morning out right by getting out of bed the right way. Instead of springing up by arching the back and jumping to the floor, start by sitting straight up with your legs out in front of you. Then swing your legs over the edge of the bed until they touch the floor. From this seated position, then, you can use your thighs and arms together, if necessary, to push yourself to a standing position.

If you have the time, it is even better to do some simple stretching even before sitting up. You can extend your arms up over your head and at the same time stretch your legs out so your spine, arms, and legs all get a good stretch before being worked for the day.

When getting out of a chair, you can use the same steps as from the sitting position step of getting out of bed. If you are sunk deeply into a soft chair or sofa, scoot to the edge so your feet are firmly planted on the floor before standing. This way you are doing more pushing with your legs, than throwing with your back for the added momentum needed to get up from that sunken position.

Getting in and out of a car can also put a strain on the spine. We tend to get in by putting one leg in, swinging our back and twisting to a seated position, then bringing the other leg in. The same is true in reverse for getting out of the car. Instead, try going in backside first. It may look a little funny, but once you are seated, then you can bring both legs around at the same time to face forward. Getting out, you can swivel the whole torso and legs simultaneously until they are on the ground outside the car, then rise to a standing position.

Shoveling

Depending on how much dirt or snow you need to move, shoveling can lead to some major back problems, not only by the weight of what is being moved, but the repetitive nature of the movement itself.

Think about how you would shovel snow from a walkway. Everyone uses one hand down low on the shovel handle, and their prominent hand up at the top. We bend at the waist, pick up the load, and then twist and throw it someplace else. This is absolutely one of the easiest ways to injure your back! The combination of weight and twisting motion are a real killer for backs. One small section of the spine carries all the weight and force of motion.

Here are some better ways to make shoveling safer for your back:

- Bend at the knees to scoop up a small amount and throw it straight ahead instead of twisting to the side. Position yourself so that you don't have to twist to unload the weight.
- Shovel deep piles of snow or dirt in layers. Don't try to lift too much weight. It not only strains the back, but can put serious stress on the heart.
- Change your grip on the shovel. By doing so, you will reduce the repetition to the same set of muscles and joints.
- Take time to stand up straight and rest. Give your back and arms a good stretch every few minutes.
- If possible, when shoveling snow, scrape small accumulations before they are deep enough to require shoveling. This way you can simply push the snow away with the shovel like a snowplow.

Backpack Syndrome

You have, no doubt, seen small children going off to school with a backpack that goes from the top of their heads, clear down to the backs of their knees. You can only imagine what those poor children are carrying that probably matches their own body weight! Backpacks themselves are not bad. In fact, they are a good way to carry a substantial load. The back and hip muscles together are a strong group. The problem with backpacks, and even heavy pocketbooks or brief cases, is how we carry them.

Whenever carrying a backpack it is important to use both shoulder straps. back to the hips. If you must carry it on one shoulder to look "cool" or for convenience, then switch shoulders often. Try to lighten the load whenever possible. Figure out what you really must carry and what can be left at home, school, or the office. For briefcases, messenger-style bags, or pocketbooks, you can put the strap over your head and across your chest to better distribute the weight. Carrying heavy bags on each side so you are balanced out with the weight will also help reduce strain on the back caused by trying to compensate for more weight on one side of the body than the other.

SLEEP POSITIONS

We really don't have much control over our sleep positions once we fall asleep. We move around in our sleep until our subconscious tells our body we are comfortable. The best way to ensure a good night's sleep, and a position that will promote a strong and healthy back, is to start out right.

The first step is to choose a mattress that supports good sleep. This will be different from one person to the next. This is often a problem with couples trying to share a bed when they have different needs and preferences for mattress firmness. New styles of beds let you have different degrees of firmness on each side and make the movement and motion of the bed mate go nearly undetected.

[176]

The sleep position that you start out in is a very personal preference. There really is no right or wrong to this decision either. The position that might be most comfortable to you could depend on different back problems you have and what areas need extra care.

For example, if you have discomfort in your shoulder or upper back, you may find it more comfortable to lie on your side and sort of hug a pillow in your arms. This relieves the pressure in the shoulder area by keeping the top shoulder in the side position propped up straight. Likewise, hip pain can be relieved by placing a pillow between the knees.

Bent knees, while lying on your back, can alleviate lower back discomfort. You can keep this position with a pillow under the knees, or by sleeping in a semi-reclined position in an adjustable bed or reclining chair.

Those who suffer from degenerative disc disease can often find comfort when sleeping on their stomachs. This stretches the spine, and opens the space between each vertebra so that there is less pain and pressure on the disc area. Relieving the facet joints is the goal for these patients as well as those with osteoarthritis.

These simple changes in the way you go about everyday movement can promote a stronger, healthier back. Just always keep in mind the three basic laws of ergonomics: to change position often, use appropriate muscle groups, and don't overextend joints.

THE ONLY EXERCISE SOME PEOPLE GET IS

JUMPING TO CONCLUSIONS, RUNNING DOWN

THEIR FRIENDS, SIDE-STEPPING

RESPONSIBILITY, AND PUSHING THEIR LUCK

~AUTHOR UNKNOWN

CONCLUSION

~14~

Chiropractic is a way of life. I hope that was evident throughout this book. It involves emotional and physical aspects of life. Chiropractic is about being well. Not just letting the numbers on a blood test tell you everything is okay, but feeling truly well and happy. Chiropractic is about diet and nutrition and about exercise and proper movement.

Above all, chiropractic is about allowing the majestic and intelligent body to perform all of the miracles of which it is innately capable. If you would like to know more about chiropractic then please visit my website at www.theactivechiro.com

REFERENCES

Chiropractic News Research; Academy of Upper Cervical Chiropractic Organizations, Inc., http://www.aucco.org/history.html

World Chiropractic Alliance, Chiropractic Basics, http://www.worldchiropracticalliance.org/consumer/basics.htm

Meeker, Haldeman, "Chiropractic: A Profession at the Crossroads of Mainstream and Alternative Medicine," Annals of Internal Medicine, 136:216-227, 2002.

Chiropractic Diagnostic Technology, by Randy Southerland, Today's Chiropractic, 2003, http://www.todayschiropractic.com/archives/may_jun_03/mj2003_feature_diag_tech.html#top.

U.S. Bureau of Labor and Statistics, Occupational Outlook, http://www.bls.gov/oco/content/ocos071.stm#top

Goertz C. Summary of 1995 ACA annual statistical survey of Chiropractic practice. J. Amer Chiropr Assoc 1996; 33 (6): 35-41.

Jenson G, et al, citing the 1993 KPMG Peat Marwick/Wayne State University Survey of 1,953 Employers.

Hurwitz EL, Coulter ID, Adams AH, Genovese BJ, Shekelle PG. Utilization of chiropractic services in the United States and Canada: 1985-1991. Am J Publ Hlth 1998;88:771-776.

Eisenberg DM, Davis RB, Ettner SL, Appel S, Wilkey S, Van Rompay M, et al, Trends in Alternative Medicine used in the United States, 1990-1997: results of a follow-up national survey. JAMA. 1998; 280:1569-75.

Hippocates Works on the Articulations; translated by Francis Adams; http://etext.library.adelaide.edu.au/h/hippocrates/h7w/articula.html

American Heritage Dictionary, http://education.yahoo.com/reference/dictionary/entry?id=c0308700

East Boston Chiropractic, Massachusetts General Laws, http://www.eastbostonchiropractic.com/definiton.htm

American Chiropractic Association, http://www.amerchiro.org/meia/growing_professsion.shtml

The Chiropractor (1[12]:10): Dr. D.D. Palmer, Allegheny, Pa., Nov. 7, 1905 as referenced in http://www.becomehealthynow.com/ebookprint.php?id=591

Chiropractic News Research; Academy of Upper Cervical Chiropractic Organizations, Inc., http://www.aucco.org/history.html.

As told at BeyondHealthy.com, http://www.becomehealthynow.com/ebookprint.php?id=591

Hypnosis, http://www.patrickdorman.com/healing_approach.htm, http://www.griffinchiropractic.net/id10.html

Types of chiropractors, methods, http://www.alternativemedicine.com/AMHome.asp?cn=Catalog&act=SearchProductXML&crt=CategoryKey=35%26StartPage=1%26PageSize=905&Style=/AMXSL/TherapyDetail.xsl

Prescription for Nutritional Healing, Third Edition, Phyllis A. Balche, CNC, James F. Balche, MD

Elderly, http://www.edgertonchiropractic.com/chiropracticforelderly.php, http://www.handsondoctor.com/pdf/research6.pdf#search='chiropractic%20for%20the%20elderly'

Acidic vs. Alkaline Foods, http://www.ctds.info/acidic-foods.html

Sharpless, SK: Susceptibility of Spinal Roots to Compression Block, NINCDS, Monograph 15, DHEW publication (NIH) 76-998, 1975, p 155-161.

Accident Analysis & Prevention. How crash severity in react impacts/influences short and long-term consequences to the neck. Vol. 32, Issue 2; March 2000; p. 187-195.

Deans, Neck Sprain –A Major Cause of Disability Following Car Accidents, pg. 10.

Holm, in The Cervical Spine, Lippincott, 1989, p. 440.

Bansley, Lord, Bogduk. Whiplash Injury: Clinical Review. Pain 58, 1994, p. 283-307.

Khan, Cook, Gargan, Bannister. Journal of Orthopedic Medicine, 21 (1), 1999, p. 22-25.

Woodward, Cook, et all (1996). "Chiropractic treatments of chronic 'whiplash'." Injury 27 (9), p. 643-645.

Freeman, Croft, Rossignol, Weaver, Reiser (1999-01). "A Review in Methodologic

Critique of the Literature Refuting Whiplash Syndrome." Spine 24(1), p. 86-89.

J Clin Epidemiol, 2000. Nov; 53(11) 1089-94.

Ryan, Neck Strain in Car Occupants: Injury Status after 6 months and Crash-Related Factors, p. 536.

McCain, Clinical Spectrum and Management of Whiplash Injuries, p. 316.

Sturezenegger, The Effect of Accident Mechanisms and Initial Findings on the Long-Term Course of Whiplash Injury, p. 446-447.

Cailliet, Neck and Arm Pain, F.A. Davis Company, 1981, p. 85.

Webb, Whiplash: Mechanisms and Patterns of Tissue Injury, Journal of Australian Chiropractors' Association, June 1985.

Murphy. Whiplash Overview 2001.

The Physician and Sports Medicine. Immobilization or early mobilization after and acute soft tissue injury? Vol. 26, No. 3; March 2000, p. 55-63.

Wall EJ, Massie JB, Kwan MK, Rydevik BL, Myers RR, Garfin SR: Experimental stretch neuropathy. Changes in nerve conduction tension. J Bone Joint Surg Br January 1992; 74 (1) p. 126-129.

Journal of Musculoskeletal Pain. A prospective study of acceleration-extension injuries following rear-end motor-vehicle crashes. Vol. 8(1/2), 200, p. 97-113.

Dietary Guidelines for Americans 2010,
http://www.health.gov/dietaryguidelines/2010.asp

ABOUT THE AUTHOR

Yaphet L Hill, obtained his undergraduate degree Florida A&M University in Tallahassee, Florida and his Doctorate of Chiropractic from Texas Chiropractic College in Pasadena, TX. Dr. Hill worked as personal trainer specializing in biomechanical dysfunction correction, muscular imbalance correction, sports specific training, and weight management. Dr. Hill utilizes certain skills ascertained as a personal trainer in his current practice in Houston, TX to evaluate and treat active and non-active individuals that suffer from acute and chronic muscle spasms, whether they be protective or segmental in origin. Muscle spasms can be caused by irritations of the nerve root, plexus, and/or nerve branch levels. Protective muscle spasms are secondary to an injury, while segmental muscle spasms occur in an uninjured segment of an injured muscle. Focusing on spinal and muscular dysfunction helps to facilitate faster recovery times from injury, while simultaneously decreasing pain levels.